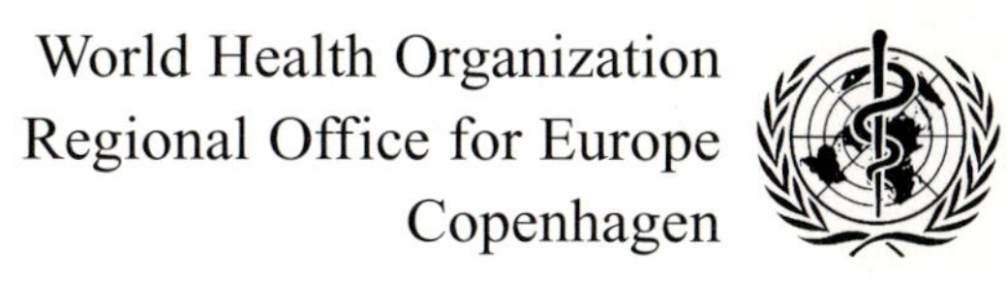

Nursing in Europe

A resource for better health

Edited by
Jane Salvage and Serge Heijnen

WHO Regional Publications, European Series, No. 74

ISBN 92 890 1338 9
ISSN 0378-2255

The designations employed and the presentation of the material in this publication do not imply the expression of any opinion whatsoever on the part of the Secretariat of the World Health Organization concerning the legal status of any country, territory, city or area or of its authorities, or concerning the delimitation of its frontiers or boundaries. The names of countries or areas used in this publication are those that obtained at the time the original language edition of the book was prepared.

The mention of specific companies or of certain manufacturers' products does not imply that they are endorsed or recommended by the World Health Organization in preference to others of a similar nature that are not mentioned. Errors and omissions excepted, the names of proprietary products are distinguished by initial capital letters.

The views expressed in this publication are those of the contributors and do not necessarily represent the decisions or the stated policy of the World Health Organization.

PRINTED IN DENMARK

WHO Library Cataloguing in Publication Data

Salvage, Jane
Nursing in Europe : a resource for better health / edited by Jane Salvage and Serge Heijnen

(WHO regional publications. European series ; No. 74)

1.Nursing 2.Midwifery 3.Europe1.Heijnen, Serge II.Title III.Series

ISBN 92 890 1338 9 (NLM Classification: WY 16)
ISSN 0378-2255

Text editing: Mary Stewart Burgher
Cover design: Sven Lund

Contents

PART II. STRATEGIES FOR ACTION

Acknowledgements

This book could not have been published without the contribution of many nurses, midwives and other health professionals throughout the WHO European Region who offered their knowledge, opinions, time and writing skills to help us understand the sociopolitical context and professional environment in which they live, work and try to fulfil their mission.

Special thanks are due not only to the contributors but also to the following people, who reviewed sections of the text: Ruth Ashton, midwifery consultant, London, United Kingdom; Gulnar Asimova, WHO collaborating centre for primary health care and nursing, Almaty, Kazakstan; Ainna Fawcett-Henesy, WHO Regional Office for Europe; Randi Mortensen, WHO collaborating centre for nursing, Copenhagen, Denmark; Bakhyt Munaidarova, former Chief Nurse, Ministry of Health, Kazakstan; Galina Perfilyeva, Head, WHO collaborating centre for nursing, Moscow, Russian Federation; Jane Robinson, Professor and Head, Department of Nursing and Midwifery Studies, University of Nottingham, United Kingdom; Tamara Sakhtanova, Chief Nurse, Ministry of Health, Kyrgyzstan; Klara Sövényi, Chief Nursing Officer, Ministry of Welfare, Hungary; and Saadet Ulker, Chief Nursing Officer, Ministry of Health, Turkey.

We are also indebted to those who helped in the production of the book: Tina Andersen and Yelena Egorenkova, formerly programme assistants, Nursing and Midwifery unit, WHO Regional Office for Europe; and Mary Stewart Burgher, Publications unit, WHO Regional Office for Europe, who offered invaluable editorial assistance.

Contributors

Ruth Ashton
Formerly Director, WHO collaborating centre for midwifery, Royal College of Midwives, London, United Kingdom

Adèle Beerling
Acting Technical Officer for Nursing, WHO Regional Office for Europe

Sally Campbell
Nurse practitioner, London, United Kingdom

Ruth Elkan
Department of Nursing and Midwifery Studies, University of Nottingham, United Kingdom

Serge Heijnen
Consultant, Health Care Policy and Administration, WHO Regional Office for Europe

Rob Keukens
Department of Nursing, State High School of Nijmegen, Netherlands

Felicity Leenders
Formerly Nursing Officer, Department of Health, London, United Kingdom

Gunnar Nielsen
Research Manager and Fellow, Danish Institute for Health and Nursing Research, Copenhagen, Denmark

Sascha Olthof
Nurse consultant, Eindhoven, Netherlands

Hans van Pernis
Department of Nursing, State High School of Nijmegen, Netherlands

Colin Ralph
Nursing consultant; formerly Registrar and Chief Executive, United Kingdom Central Council for Nursing, Midwifery and Health Visiting, London, United Kingdom

Jane Robinson
Professor and Head, Department of Nursing and Midwifery Studies, University of Nottingham, United Kingdom

Jane Salvage
Formerly Regional Adviser for Nursing and Midwifery, WHO Regional Office for Europe; now Editor, *Nursing times*, London, United Kingdom

Alison Tierney
Reader, Department of Nursing Studies, University of Edinburgh, United Kingdom

Abbreviations

ACTN	Advisory Committee on the Training of Nurses (EU)
CCEE	countries of central and eastern Europe
CE	Council of Europe
EC	European Community
EFTA	European Free Trade Association
EU	European Union
EUROQUAN	European Nursing Quality Network
GDP	gross domestic product
GP	general medical practitioner
ICD-10	International Statistical Classification of Diseases and Related Health Problems, tenth revision
ICM	International Confederation of Midwives
ICN	International Council of Nurses
ICNP	international classification for nursing practice
ILO	International Labour Organisation
LEMON	Learning Materials on Nursing project (WHO)
LINK	Leaders in Nursing Network (WHO)
NIS	newly independent states of the former USSR
NNA	national nursing association
NMA	national midwifery association
OECD	Organisation for Economic Co-operation and Development
PCN	Standing Committee of Nurses of the European Union
PHC	primary health care
PSI	Public Services International
UNICEF	United Nations Children's Fund
WENR	Workgroup of European Nurse Researchers

Foreword

What is the most important resource for health that a European country has today? Countries would give different answers to this question, but all of them would put the work of nurses very high on the list – and rightfully so! The sheer number of the profession is close to 5 million in the 50 countries of the WHO European Region. They serve the Region's 850 million people, who live in an area bordered by Greenland in the west, the Mediterranean Sea in the south, and the Pacific shores of the Russian Federation in the east. Nurses are not a homogeneous group: large differences are found in the roles they play, the tasks they perform, the training they receive, the status they have in society and the remuneration they get for their work. Taken together, however, they comprise a formidable workforce that provides some of the most essential services to keep people healthy, to take care of the ill and the injured, and to nurse the frail and elderly throughout the Region.

In many, if not most, European countries, these health professionals unfortunately do not get the recognition they deserve, or the working facilities they need to carry out their unique function in our health care systems.

The WHO Regional Office for Europe has had a very strong programme in nursing for many years, because it believes that only a well trained community nurse can really be the first line of defence of the primary health care system. The model that WHO foresees is the one that emerged in 1988 from WHO's First European Conference on Nursing in Vienna, by which a nurse is responsible for providing a broad community-based service (including lifestyle counselling, diagnosis of health problems and home care for the sick, frail and elderly) in addition to the important nursing function in the hospital sector. In spite of intensive work since the Conference, however, nurses are still far from that situation in many Member States. There is an urgent need for countries thoroughly to revise their policies, infrastructures and training programmes for nursing to make them compatible with the WHO models.

The nursing and midwifery programme in the Regional Office is working hard to attain these objectives. In view of the serious problems related to nursing in most of the countries of the Region, WHO has concentrated on helping those countries in the most difficult situations. To help these countries and the other Member States of the Region, as well as to improve countries' nursing policies and services, the first requirement is an understanding of the current situation. This will provide a sound foundation for new initiatives and indicate the urgent needs for reform. WHO's European Nursing and Midwifery unit prepared this book to meet these needs. The first of its kind, it gives a thorough overview of the current state of nursing and midwifery in Europe, and contains a wealth of extremely useful information for nurses, their professional organizations, ministries of health, ministries of education and other bodies that are interested in promoting better health and improving health services in the European Region. A previous book produced by our Nursing and Midwifery unit – Nursing in action *– became a best-seller, and no doubt this book will follow in its footsteps.*

J.E. Asvall
WHO Regional Director for Europe

Introduction

Jane Salvage

The 50 Member States of the WHO European Region cover a huge area stretching from the west coast of Greenland to the Pacific coast of the Russian Federation and from the Arctic to the Mediterranean Sea. For WHO, Europe is a loose geographical definition, since it incorporates all the newly independent states (NIS) of the former USSR, including those in central Asia. After the Second World War, the map of Europe was clearly redrawn and its borders and systems remained fairly stable until the unprecedented changes in the countries of central and eastern Europe (CCEE) and the USSR in the late 1980s. These changes were accompanied by severe social and economic problems, and armed conflict in many of the countries. The social cost of change continues to be high and it is impossible to predict where all the changes will lead. Moreover, they have had a major and as yet immeasurable impact on the rest of Europe. Meanwhile, the European Union has expanded and continues to grapple with the issue of extending membership to eastern Europe.

That is the backdrop to the issues raised in this book. The last publication from the Nursing and Midwifery unit of the WHO Regional Office for Europe, *Nursing in action (1)*, described visions, goals and policy guidelines that had mostly been developed during the 1980s. The changes in Europe had barely begun when the first WHO European Conference on Nursing, which laid down the framework for nursing development in the Region, took place in Vienna in 1988 *(2)*. This provoked some hard questions as the new Europe of the 1990s took shape. Was the Vienna Declaration and subsequent WHO and other international guidance relevant only to western Europe? Could WHO be sure that those visions, goals and guidelines were still useful? This book shows how the Nursing and Midwifery unit at the Regional Office examined these questions in partnership with Member States, what conclusions were reached, and what policies and programmes were initiated in response to the priority needs expressed by the countries.

The Need for Good Information

There was one immediate obstacle to progress. In 1988, the European Region had 32 Member States; in the 1990s, it has 50. Not only were contacts and relationships lacking with many of the new countries, but also little was known about them. Without better information, WHO could neither assess the situation accurately nor respond to countries' requests for help with nursing development. Furthermore, the countries themselves usually lacked much of this information, for a variety of reasons. The Nursing and Midwifery unit therefore spent four years collecting data from every country and feeding it into country nursing and midwifery profiles, of which there are now 46. We can now look comprehensively at the real picture of nursing and midwifery across the whole Region, make comparisons and map trends – the first time such a task has been attempted. This book gives the first full description of the current situation in nursing and midwifery in Europe, and the beginnings of an analysis. Now that WHO has established this baseline, further analysis and trend-spotting can be undertaken, and become easier and more accurate.

The data presented in Part I should be interpreted in the light of the overall social, political and health context of the Region. The population of Europe is around 850 million and expected to rise slowly. Fertility rates have fallen, marriage is becoming less frequent and divorce is increasing. The population continues to age, with a notable increase in people aged 60–79; the economically active population is also aging. Cultural, social, political and economic factors are all very diverse, making generalizations about the Region and about nursing fraught with difficulty. Such generalization becomes a little more meaningful, however, if the Region is divided into subregions for analytical purposes, as we have done here.

Our data show huge variations in nursing and midwifery across the Region. In particular they show a wide gap in the quality of care between west and east, caused partly by the crisis now engulfing the health care systems of eastern countries but also by their historical neglect of nursing and midwifery. Indeed, as the recent WHO Expert Committee on Nursing Practice observed, there is no direct correlation between the socioeconomic condition of a country and the scope of nursing practice *(3)*. Regardless of the state of development of nursing services, a variety of factors impedes their effective delivery in many countries. These factors include the exclusion of nurses from policy-making and decision-making at all levels of the health care system, shortages of well trained nurses relative to needs, insufficient financial support and the undervaluing of nursing, with its concomitant subordination to medicine. The position is further complicated by continuing gender discrimination. Nursing everywhere is women's work and shares the characteristics of other female-dominated occupations: low pay, low status, poor working conditions, few prospects for promotion and poor education.

Nevertheless, awareness is growing of the need to examine the role of nursing. Starting points and initial conditions differ widely between countries, and so do the responses. It is possible, however, to distinguish some emerging trends. First, nurses, like all other health care providers, are under increasing pressure to prove they are good value for money. This has spurred greater efforts to measure the outcomes of nursing interventions (particularly in the United Kingdom and northern Europe). Second, interest is growing in nursing education, where key issues include the review and reorientation of the curriculum to primary health care (PHC); the development of new programmes, especially in higher education; the training of nurse educators; the provision of high-quality education materials; the development of continuing education schemes; and the forging of closer links between education and services. Third, attitudes towards the position of nursing in society and its role in health care are slowly changing. The perception of nursing as a low-status occupation requiring minimal training, and the associated undervaluation of humanistic, psychosocial care are beginning to alter, although the process is very slow and uneven.

Nursing, Health for All and Health Care Reform

In 1984, the WHO Regional Committee for Europe adopted a framework for public health policy, setting out the improvements needed to secure health for all and describing strategies for achieving them through healthier lifestyles, improvements in the environment and the provision of high-quality health services. These strategies, it was proposed, could be implemented using a target approach: 38 health for all targets and related indicators *(4)*. The targets were intended to support the formulation and implementation of health policies in Member States, and the indicators would enable comparisons between countries and the monitoring of trends. The endorsement of this framework by all

Member States was very encouraging, and health policy development took a big step forward. As yet, however, there has been no real progress towards the primary target for health for all: equity. The health gap between the northern and western and the central and eastern parts of the Region is actually widening as health improves in the former and deteriorates in the latter. There is also a widening health gap within countries, related to income. Closing these gaps by improving the health of particular population groups, at least to the level of the differences that existed at the beginning of the 1970s, is today's major challenge.

In the Declaration of Alma-Ata, emanating from the 1978 International Conference on Primary Health Care *(5)*, WHO Member States had already advocated the development of PHC as the key strategy for the attainment of health for all. Today, virtually all the countries of western Europe have adopted policy goals that shift health care delivery towards PHC and closer to the community, workplace and home, with less dependence on institutional care. In reality, however, progress has been uneven and slow. In addition, the Conference urged governments to:

> give high priority to the full utilization of human resources by defining the technical role, supportive skills, and attitudes required for each category of health worker according to the functions that need to be carried out to ensure effective primary health care…

This implies that nursing should be a key component of PHC, and an essential vehicle for health for all.

The main resource of every health care system is the personnel who work in it. Staff pay is a major budget item and staff control most of the other expenditure, but money is not the whole story. The quality of the contribution of each person, from the top manager to the floor cleaner, is central to success or failure. In the long run, the achievements of any health care system are primarily influenced not by the choice of structure or funding mechanism, important as these are, but by how well the system develops, motivates and deploys its staff. Major reform of nursing and midwifery should therefore be an important aspect of health care transition. Although it does not grab the headlines like other measures, such as the commercialization of medicine or the emergency supply of drugs, such reform could arguably have a greater long-term impact on health services.

Health care reform is a major issue in nearly all the countries of the Region. In the CCEE and NIS there is much debate about how far the Soviet model of health care, which dominated these countries to a greater or lesser extent, can or should be adapted to new needs. Formidable problems are emerging from the efforts to achieve change quickly –often too quickly and with incomplete understanding of the policy options, not to mention poor resources. These countries' concerns about how to find the right balance between public and private health care provision echo throughout the Region, where many if not most countries – faced with apparently endless needs and diminishing resources – are experimenting with different approaches to the financing of health care systems. This can create interesting innovations, but an overriding concern with financing and structure – which tends to focus on acute hospitals and the role of doctors – is detrimental to the development of PHC. Unfortunately, nursing and midwifery are not seen as very important in these debates; although many countries are aware of the need to tackle such issues as staff recruitment, retention and education, and the quality of care, these topics are not in general high on the political agenda.

Nurses and midwives, however, are fundamental to health care in Europe. They comprise the largest single group of health professionals in the Region and therefore exert great influence – even if indirectly. (If the reform agenda fails to inspire the nursing and midwifery professions, its long-term success must be doubtful or even impossible.) Around 5 million people work in the nursing services of the 50 Member States, half of them in the CCEE and NIS. They promote health, prevent disease and provide care. The World Bank has identified nursing and midwifery personnel as the most cost-effective resource for delivering high-quality public health and clinical packages. These factors link nursing's fortunes much more closely to the reform of health care systems, with all that that implies for interactive impact, than is usually recognized.

This presents a major challenge to every country's health services and especially to those of the CCEE and NIS, where there is mounting evidence of failure to train staff adequately for their roles or to deploy them effectively, of oversupply of some staff and shortages of others, of very poor wages and working conditions, and of low morale. The effects of these problems will become increasingly acute as people gain more freedom to move within and between countries, and to sell their scarce skills in a more competitive labour market. Plans for health care reform are unlikely to succeed in the absence of concurrent plans for the best use of human resources for health. To put the case at its most extreme, no system can work properly if its best staff have left. A comprehensive national health care plan must include these issues as part of its strategy, and tackle them at the same time.

Effectiveness: health outcomes and health care

A surprisingly large proportion of the work of health care professionals – doctors, nurses, physiotherapists and others – is ineffective and even harmful. This statement is supported by evidence from many countries, including the United Kingdom and the United States, and is probably true of many if not most other countries. Even where clear scientific evidence exists, staff continue to use dangerous or outdated techniques that injure patients and waste money. The content of professional health work must be strictly scrutinized to ensure that it is appropriate and effective. Relevant tools include quality assurance systems, clinical audit, clinical research, strategies for research implementation and continuing education for professionals. The principles underlying these techniques are relevant to any health care system, and the tools can be adapted according to its stage of development.

Peer review of the effectiveness of health care interventions can be facilitated by the development of strong, independent professional institutions that derive their authority from their commitment to serving the public. This is not synonymous with traditional, élitist professionalism, but points to a new model of professionalism that emphasizes working in partnership with patients and populations.

Efficiency: making the best use of personnel

Workforce planning is an essential component of an effective health care strategy. It is needed to ensure that the profile of the health care labour force is designed to meet people's needs for health care, and that appropriate steps are then taken to match the supply of staff to the demand. This is a complex exercise involving at least the following elements:

- identifying health care needs and how the service aims to meet them;
- clarifying the role and functions of each group of staff, including doctors, nurses, other therapists, auxiliary staff and other support workers;
- reviewing education programmes to ensure that staff are properly prepared for their roles;
- planning the best mix of grades and skills in the health care team, based on the agreed role and function, as well as experience, of each member;
- determining the number of staff needed in each grade and regulating labour supply (recruitment and training) accordingly; and

- offering incentives (such as more pay, better working conditions, and opportunities for development) to attract and retain high-quality staff.

Management: planning for the future

Good management is crucial to success. People with management capabilities must be identified and trained to create a core of managers with modern management skills – a combination of leadership and administrative expertise. They may be doctors, nurses or other health professionals (few of whom can automatically be good managers without extra training and in-service development), experienced managers from other sectors or specially recruited general management trainees. In addition, the management style of the organization is critical: evidence suggests that the most successful organizations are those that motivate their staff, reward them for good work and involve them in decision-making. Good management therefore includes paying attention to organizational development and to creating incentives for all staff.

One aspect of organizational development that is of special current relevance to the CCEE and NIS is the management of change. Professional and management training needs to accept change as the norm, and to give people the capacities to respond effectively in terms of the structures in which they work, the patterns of their work, the tools they use and their responses to new evidence. Organizations and individuals that are unable to be flexible and sensitive to change, and to handle its impact on people and institutions, will fail to thrive in the Europe of the future.

Power sharing: the devolution of responsibility and authority

Decentralization is a strong theme of today's health care reforms. If it is to have any beneficial effect, it means devolving authority and responsibility to the lowest possible levels in the health service. Whether they are clinical, administrative or support staff, people must have the authority to make decisions on the issues that lie within their competence. In return for giving them this authority and expecting them to be responsible and accountable for what they do, the organization must offer them proper training and support, and respect the integrity of their decisions.

Power must be shared not simply among health service staff but also between them and the users of services. Participatory care is essential for effectiveness and efficiency, not just a luxury for consumer-oriented societies. It means involving citizens directly in every stage of health care, from service planning to evaluation. It means offering them genuine choices based on full information, and evolving new styles of professional behaviour based on doing things with patients rather than to them. After all, people should really be considered not as consumers of health services but as producers of their own health. Ultimately, the major human resource of any health care system is its citizens.

Visions, Policies and Actions

Part I of this book paints a picture of the current situation. Part II moves on to explore some visions of nursing's future role, and some policies and actions designed to turn those visions into reality. It focuses particularly on ideas and tools developed via WHO in the 1990s. In fact, the nursing professions were the first to scrutinize their practice and respond to health for all in the context of public health. As the WHO Regional Director for Europe has commented, delivering an integrated, health-promoting, preventive and curative service to the people of the Region will require a strong nursing team working in close collaboration with general medical practitioners and other health and social personnel at community level. In fact, the implementation of health for all policy will not be possible without such a new role for and input from nursing.

This vision cannot become reality without strong nursing leadership, which is explored in Part II in relation to the linked issues of national policies and strategies for nursing and midwifery, and the role of nurses and midwives in government. These topics have been a particular focus of the Nursing and Midwifery unit of the WHO Regional Office for Europe in the 1990s, and have been tackled in innovative ways. Leadership without knowledge is meaningless, however, and the programme has therefore also focused on making good nursing information of all kinds readily available. The WHO LEMON (LEarning Materials On Nursing) project was designed to start filling this knowledge gap in the CCEE and NIS, but also aims to build capacity in countries and individuals, as described in Part II. As this part of the book draws heavily on WHO work, it may be helpful to set out here some of the assumptions on which the regional programme is based.

- Health care is an important determinant of health, although by no means the most important.
- The PHC approach is the key to maximizing the impact of health services, and to improving the quality of nursing.

- Nursing staff comprise the largest group of people working in any health service, so that their influence on the quality of the service is extremely important, though largely unrecognized.
- Nurses (as professionals and also as women) are marginalized by men, doctors and governments, so that nursing development has to be partly remedial work to ensure that the effects of this marginalization (such as poor education and the lack of top posts) are counteracted – in other words, to bring nurses on to a level playing field with the rest.
- The best way for WHO to influence these factors and advocate needed change is to empower nurses themselves to tackle the issues more effectively.

Certain assumptions about change also underlie the programme; the factors that drive an effective change process are:

- a vision of what should be achieved
- a strong value base
- a strategy to give a clear direction and priorities for action
- an action plan
- accountability, with designated roles and responsibilities
- leadership
- talk, talk and more talk, to review and modify as circumstances demand openness.

The change process will only succeed in the long term if it is based on valuing every human being equally, and therefore uses democratic and participatory processes at every stage. Indeed, the journey to change is as important as the destination. A good change process is essential but it still may not succeed, owing to both predictable and unpredictable factors; human life and behaviour are by definition chaotic. The entry point for change varies according to circumstances but always depends on the success of agents of change in creating a critical mass of support. The programme therefore aims to create or use a variety of entry points, ranging from national leadership (national action plans for nursing) to groups of activists combining personal and positional power (the LEMON country groups) to grassroots clinical projects. This flexibility is essential. The programme staff believe that technical knowledge is important but cannot be forced on people; they learn when they are ready. Much of what the staff do is designed to stimulate people to seek knowledge, as well as to help them to find the information they need. The approach therefore balances the human and technical input. Finally, as part of a development agency, the staff know they can exert great influence by modelling the processes they encourage others to use. They practise what they preach.

Shaping the Future

Part III of the book, on work in progress, is rather different. Its chapters on PHC nursing and measuring nursing highlight areas where further thinking is required, and offer some ideas for debate. Unlike the policies and projects featured in Part II, they have not been widely discussed among the European nursing community, although they have been developed with care, a sound knowledge base and peer review during the drafting. PHC nursing in Europe needs new thinking because, although it is not new, the context in which it should be practised is and, like the health care systems of which it is part, is changing daily. In addition, the vision of the Declaration of Alma-Ata and the way it is pursued need to be revisited and refreshed to inspire and support new generations of health workers and citizens. Measuring nursing, as mentioned earlier, is a growing trend that relates more pragmatically to the same question of how to reach defined goals. The search is on for ways to assess nursing efficiency and effectiveness. Informatics is one area of this in which nurses are gaining expertise; they are also exploring its relevance to nursing development.

A Note on Terminology

For convenience, nursing and nurse are used in this book as general terms. Terminology and definitions vary from country to country, and indeed direct translation of the terms is sometimes impossible. "Nurses" should be understood to mean all health workers doing nursing-related work, including nurses, midwives and feldshers. In some CCEE and NIS, this also means those doing physiotherapy and other tasks; these occupations are not regarded as distinct professions owing to the poorly differentiated division of labour. Some countries regard nursing and midwifery as one profession, while others have separate regulatory, education and professional bodies for the two occupations. In using the term nursing, no assumptions are made or implied about nursing's relationship to midwifery. The need for leaders to promote a strategic, knowledge-based approach to development is just as crucial in midwifery as in nursing, but whether this development takes place jointly or separately is a matter for each country to decide. Either way, it is in the interest of both groups to define their goals and to work together on the many areas of mutual concern. The same point applies to other groups, such as feldshers.

Conclusion

This book offers a range of new information, visions, policies and ideas for action. It is based on the inspiration and experiences of nursing and midwifery leaders throughout the European Region. We hope it will inspire you to join in the quest for health for all.

References

1. Salvage, J., ed. *Nursing in action. Strengthening nursing and midwifery to support health for all.* Copenhagen, WHO Regional Office for Europe, 1993 (WHO Regional Publications, European Series, No. 48).
2. *European Conference on Nursing*. Copenhagen, WHO Regional Office for Europe, 1989.
3. *Nursing practice. Report of a WHO Expert Committee.* Geneva, World Health Organization, 1996 (WHO Technical Report Series, No. 860).
4. *Health for all targets. The health policy for Europe*. Copenhagen, WHO Regional Office for Europe, 1993 (European Health for All Series, No. 4).
5. *Alma-Ata 1978: Primary health care.* Geneva, World Health Organization, 1978 ("Health for All" Series, No. 1).

Part I
Nursing in Europe: the Current Situation

1

Introduction

Jane Salvage & Serge Heijnen

This study is part of a WHO initiative to collect, analyse and disseminate essential data on nursing and midwifery. The massive changes to the map of Europe and their subsequent impact on health and health care indicated the need for an organized database on nursing, as did requests for information from nurses and others, particularly those in new Member States. The Nursing and Midwifery unit at the WHO Regional Office for Europe had already collected much raw data on nursing, but some were not readily accessible and some were missing. The health for all database and other programmes in the Regional Office had little information relevant to nursing or midwifery, making it statistically invisible.

Inquiries confirmed that many nurses working in ministries of health and other nursing leaders, especially in the CCEE and the NIS, did not have access to useful data. Data often did not exist, and nursing leaders sometimes mistrusted official statistics. Key information on workforce planning, education reform, project development and many other activities was hard to find. The Soviet system in particular had emphasized the collection of statistics, but these were frequently inaccurate and rarely fed back to service providers in any meaningful way. This lack of information meant that nursing leaders were denied the means to participate in the powerful processes of communication, and that their contribution to policy formulation was marginalized. Not only the countries themselves but also the agencies charged with assisting them, including WHO, were working in the dark. This made the compilation of the present type of report almost impossible. The international exchange of knowledge, the sharing of experiences to stimulate awareness of potential solutions, and sound knowledge of the state of health care in countries are essential for an understanding of nursing, and enable nursing leaders to make a positive contribution to health care policy.

The Regional Office Nursing and Midwifery unit therefore started a project in 1992 to collect, review and disseminate essential data.

This study of nursing in Europe is carried out in parallel with, and contributes to, an initiative by WHO headquarters to monitor progress on implementing World Health Assembly resolution WHA45.5 on strengthening nursing and midwifery in support of strategies for health for all *(1)*. The starting point of this global study was a questionnaire to all Member States to obtain essential information, processed and analysed to assist them and WHO to assess the current situation, to provide input to policy changes and to promote nursing and midwifery as essential health services. Studies to find ways of measuring the impact on health of direct nursing interventions are planned in selected countries. The participation of the European programme in this project and its own evaluation process both contributes to and is strengthened by the global experience. In addition, the proposed global research will attempt to determine whether the implementation of resolutions has any relationship to health and economic indicators, and what needs to be done to help Member States develop policies to implement these resolutions.

The European study began with the decision to produce a profile of nursing and midwifery in each of the CCEE and NIS. As time went by, other countries requested their own profiles and the project was extended to the whole Region. The first step was to draw up a draft minimum data list for structuring the collection of information. This and a sample profile were assessed in 1992 by a group of nursing leaders from nine countries, east and west. They liked the form used (and suggested some changes) and thought the profiles would provide them with a comprehensive planning base: a powerful source of information to help them analyse nursing in their countries and prepare national action plans, project proposals and plans for resource mobilization. Since then, data have been collected and processed for all Member States using the minimum data list. The profiles archive the information held by the Regional Office and countries, providing a system that makes information readily available and easily updated (resources permitting). The compilation of the profiles is an interactive process; it makes progress slow and labour intensive, but the involvement of nursing leaders is crucial.

The information collected in the draft profiles was collated and analysed, resulting in a first raw mapping. Experts from several European countries and different nursing specialties contributed to the analysis, especially in areas where the information was still insufficient, or where a trend or positive development in nursing's contribution to health for all could be made more visible. Part I of this book is the result. It describes the current state of nursing, the issues nurses grapple with, often in very difficult circumstances, and various ways in which they are preparing themselves to assume a role as autonomous practitioners able to work in the hospital and community (and thereby actively work towards health for all targets 28 and 29 *(2)*)[1]. By no means all the wealth of information in the profiles is reproduced in this book; individual country profiles can be obtained from the Regional Office on request. A summary of all the profiles as they stood at January 1995 has been produced as a separate document, to be read in conjunction with this chapter by those who require more detail *(5)*.

Objectives of the Study

The aim of this study of nursing in Europe is to support European nurses' efforts to improve the health and wellbeing of patients and communities. Its more specific objectives are:

- to make existing information on nursing and midwifery readily available to Member States and WHO;
- to analyse the state of the art of nursing in the European Region and evaluate progress, including making comparisons between countries and identifying trends;
- to contribute to research-based health development in Europe and to stimulate the creation of strategies for nursing;
- to contribute data and ideas to a variety of WHO programmes and initiatives in the European Region;
- to contribute to implementation of World Health Assembly resolutions and other global initiatives on nursing; and
- to make nursing in Europe more visible.

It may act as a catalyst for change and convince others of the need for nursing development, supporting the arguments of national nursing leaders with facts, ideas and recommendations. This study is the first of its kind to be carried out in the European Region. Its range, focus and intent will interest many people, including health policy-makers at all levels, researchers, health care and nursing organizations, and anyone concerned with the state of nursing in Europe. It puts nursing and midwifery in Europe on the map.

---

[1] The health for all nurse is one who contributes to achieving the goals of health for all. The mission, role and functions are comprehensively described in the Vienna Declaration *(3)* and subsequent WHO publications, notably *Nursing in action (4)*.

This mainly descriptive study is important, but "harder" measures of progress are also needed. It is notoriously difficult to produce valid, reliable, sensitive and specific indicators of the impact of different types of health policy and health care delivery. Nevertheless, it might be possible to develop some criteria to help assess progress in nursing development at the national and international levels; at present such indicators are poorly developed or nonexistent. There is plenty of conventional wisdom about what combination of factors promotes good nursing and midwifery practice – ranging from high-quality education to the existence of a professional regulatory framework – but there is relatively little hard evidence. Proxy measures would help WHO and countries to run more effective programmes and target more precisely where efforts should be directed. Regional and subregional trends could be mapped and analysed. Indicators measured at intervals of several years would tell countries how they were progressing, and provide material for fruitful comparisons.

Some ambitious initiatives are exploring outcome indicators for nursing practice. The WHO Global Advisory Group on Nursing and Midwifery is leading this at the international level with a project to define indicators for monitoring nursing's contribution to health for all. Similar projects are under way at the national level, mostly aiming to define nursing elements in national health databases. For example, a valuable initiative to explore the complex relationship between nursing input and health outcomes comes from the Canadian Nurses Association and the Alberta Association of Registered Nurses *(6)*. They are supporting the development of a minimum data set to ensure the entry, accessibility and retrievability of nursing data. The aim is to identify measurable indicators related to client status, reflecting the phenomena for which nurses provide care in relation to the cultural status of clients; nursing interventions, referring to purposeful and deliberate (direct and indirect) interventions that affect health; client outcome, or the client's status at a defined point following intervention; and nursing intensity, which refers to the amount and type of nursing resources used to provide care. Once identified, "health information: nursing components" will be a minimum set of items of information, with uniform definitions and categories concerning the specific dimensions of professional nursing, that meets the information needs of multiple data users in the health care system.

In the European Region, important examples of work to make nursing statistically visible are the TELENURSING and TELENURSE projects funded by the European Union (EU). A detailed description of the objectives, activities and expected outcomes is provided in Chapter 8.

A Word of Warning

The original purpose of the profiles was to provide readily accessible information. The work was not funded as a research project, although the Nursing and Midwifery unit took scientific research criteria into account when possible. Data were collected from official sources and supplemented by informal findings. While they are as reliable as they could be made, it is impossible to guarantee accuracy for several reasons. These include inadequate resources and infrastructures for the collection of information. Terminology differs widely, making direct comparisons difficult. Societies and health systems are in transition in many countries, and data in some profiles may already be out of date. Further, any attempt to describe the work, roles, education, management and so on of nearly 5 million nursing personnel, in an area as historically, culturally, geographically, economically and sociopolitically diverse as the European Region, must have many shortcomings. This study should be read with these warnings in mind. Nevertheless, the data should be accepted as reasonable for the purposes for which they were collected; and their quantity and quality are in general sufficiently robust and sensitive, despite some gaps, for analytical purposes.

Finally, readers may note one particularly large gap in this study: a description of the actual daily work of nurses and midwives. Rules, regulations, laws and ideals concerning practice can be described fairly readily, but capturing the reality of the nurse's work is much more difficult. Attempts to elicit this type of data from countries have not been successful, perhaps because the official version and the daily reality are rather far apart in many countries, and countries understandably wish to present themselves in the best light. (Interestingly, the countries that have historically been the most secretive in the Region now tend to be much more open than the others about their nursing problems.) Without a detailed understanding of the actual work, however, changes are difficult to make. Much can be inferred by reading between the lines of this study, but further research on this, based on direct observation of and reporting by practitioners, is badly needed *(7)*.

References

1. *Handbook of resolutions and decisions of the World Health Assembly and the Executive Board, Vol. III, 3rd ed. (1985–1992)*. Geneva, World Health Organization, 1993.
2. *Health for all targets. The health policy for Europe.* Copenhagen,

WHO Regional Office for Europe, 1993 (European Health for All Series, No. 4).
3. *European Conference on Nursing. Report on a WHO meeting.* Copenhagen, WHO Regional Office for Europe, 1989.
4. SALVAGE, J., ED. *Nursing in action. Strengthening nursing and midwifery to support health for all.* Copenhagen, WHO Regional Office for Europe, 1993 (WHO Regional Publications, European Series, No. 48).
5. *Summary of country profiles on nursing and midwifery in Member States of the WHO European Region.* Copenhagen, WHO Regional Office for Europe, 1997 (document ICP/DLVR 04 01 01).
6. *Papers from the Alberta Association of Registered Nurses health information: nursing components working session.* Edmonton, Alberta Association of Registered Nurses, 1993.
7. SALVAGE, J. Raising the nursing profile: the case of the invisible nurse. *World health statistics quarterly*, **46**(3): 170–176 (1993).

2

Nursing and midwifery in Europe

Jane Salvage & Serge Heijnen

Developments in nursing and midwifery in Europe are taking place in the context of growing demands for accessible, affordable, high-quality health care and a recognition that health and disease are everyone's responsibility. Successes have been achieved in improving health, but the aging of the population, the AIDS pandemic and the recurrence of some communicable diseases are placing new demands on health care services. Recent social phenomena, such as urbanization and large-scale migration, have the same effect. At the same time, responses to these growing demands for health care are influenced by scarcity of resources and by ideological decisions about the role of the welfare state. Services delivered by nurses are increasingly perceived as having huge but unfulfilled potential for attaining improvements in health and containing costs.

This chapter provides an overview of the current state of nursing in Europe by summarizing and analysing the nursing and midwifery profiles for 45 WHO European Member States, supplemented by key research papers and policy documents on nursing development. Sufficient information could not be collected on some countries: Bosnia and Herzegovina, Luxembourg, Monaco, San Marino and the Federal Republic of Yugoslavia (Serbia and Montenegro). Furthermore, throughout this chapter and in its conclusions, the current situation is compared to the goals formulated at the first WHO European Conference on Nursing *(1)* and other key global and European guidelines and statements. The study is intended not to be complete and final, but to give greater impetus to an existing movement.

The subsections in this chapter echo the headings of the profiles' minimum data set and are milestones for nursing development: policy,

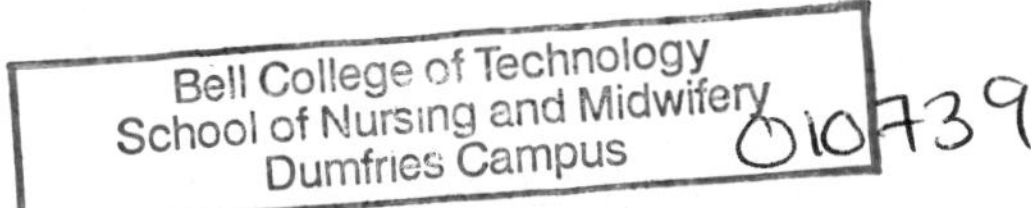

leadership, regulatory frameworks, role of the nurse, terms and conditions, human resources, education, research and quality of care, professional organizations and communications. They create the framework for practice and define the areas in which strategies need to be developed and implemented. The importance of each milestone is shown by a survey undertaken by the International Council of Nurses (ICN) in 1993–1994 *(2)*. European national nursing associations (NNAs) reported that the top five priority areas in nursing were, in descending order, education, legislation, health policy, working conditions and standards of care. In addition, nursing research and nursing leadership were ranked in the top ten. As described earlier, difficulties remain in identifying causal relationships between one or more of the milestones and the effective delivery of nursing services, and particularly population health or patient wellbeing. The presentation of these milestones does not imply any judgement on their importance. Developments and services are at various stages within and between countries, and appropriate strategic action has to be identified in accordance with the situation in each country and at each administrative level. This undoubtedly leads to different priorities.

Data are presented in the same sequence under each heading. First, the topic and its relevance to nursing development are discussed. Key statements and recommendations are mentioned. Then follows a description of the current situation in the CCEE, NIS and western Europe, or a combination of these subregions, with some country examples and cross-references to the statements mentioned. These subregions are used as an analytical framework to help organize the mass of data on nearly 50 countries. Very broadly speaking, the countries in each subregion share many common characteristics with regard to history, political systems and current social and economic changes.

For the purposes of this study, the CCEE comprise Albania, Bosnia and Herzegovina, Bulgaria, Croatia, the Czech Republic, Hungary, Poland, Romania, Slovakia, Slovenia, The Former Yugoslav Republic of Macedonia and the Federal Republic of Yugoslavia (Serbia and Montenegro). The NIS comprise Armenia, Azerbaijan, Belarus, Estonia, Georgia, Kazakstan, Kyrgyzstan, Latvia, Lithuania, the Republic of Moldova, the Russian Federation, Tajikistan, Turkmenistan, Ukraine and Uzbekistan.

For convenience, the remaining subregion is called western Europe. The term is not geographically accurate but an alternative is difficult to find; not all the countries in this group belong to the Organisation for Economic Co-operation and Development (OECD) or the EU. This group comprises the rest of the European Region: Austria, Belgium, Denmark, Finland, France, Germany, Greece, Iceland, Ireland, Israel, Italy, Luxembourg, Malta, Monaco, the Netherlands, Norway, Portugal, San Marino, Spain, Sweden, Switzerland, Turkey and the United Kingdom.

Policy

Prevailing political, cultural and socioeconomic conditions have always had a significant impact on the delivery of nursing services. Nursing practice, however, has shown a consistent commitment to change through flexible and responsive development *(3)*. As a result, nursing is now a key activity in every practice setting imaginable. In some countries it ranges from carrying out high-technology investigations in academic hospitals to providing the whole range of PHC services in remote regions. In most countries, however, these diverse nursing roles have not developed in a planned or systematic way. The ad hoc development of nursing practice, both to meet the population's needs and to help contain costs, has made it difficult for policy-makers, planners and nurses themselves to describe the nature and scope of nursing and, at times, to differentiate it from the practice of other health workers.

The challenge for nursing is to provide appropriate and cost-effective forms of care based on health needs and within the context of a country's political, economic, social and cultural resources. A national strategic planning process for nursing, with input from nurses and others, can identify the vision for the future and set out priorities for action in a national action plan for nursing. Ideally, this strategy is integrated into all decision-making processes relating to health policy and planning, to ensure that the entire nursing workforce is working towards national health goals *(1)*.

The desire of nurses for greater influence on national health policy is supported by the 1977 International Labour Organisation (ILO) Convention 149 on nursing *(4)*; Article 2 explicitly states that:

> 1. Each Member which ratifies this Convention shall adopt and apply, in a manner appropriate to national conditions, a policy concerning nursing services and nursing personnel designed, within the framework of a general health programme, where such a programme exists, and within the resources available for health care as a whole, to provide the quantity and quality of nursing care necessary for attaining the highest possible level of health for the population.

2. In particular, it shall take the necessary measures to provide nursing personnel with –
(a) education and training appropriate to the exercise of their function; and
(b) employment and working conditions, including career prospects and remuneration, which are likely to attract persons to the profession and retain them in it.

3. The policy mentioned in paragraph 1 of this Article shall be formulated in consultation with the employers' and workers' organisations concerned, where such organisations exist.

4. This policy shall be co-ordinated with policies relating to other aspects of health care and to other workers in the field of health, in consultation with the employers' and workers' organisations concerned.

Several WHO global and European meetings in the early 1990s reinforced the importance of a strategic approach to nursing development in support of health for all. Countries are at various stages in the development of national action plans, and the scope and purpose of these plans also vary. A few countries, like the United Kingdom, have developed comprehensive strategies, including targets for practice, education, management and research. Others take a more narrowly focused starting point; for example, Greece proposes starting with the establishment of a national council for nursing development. In addition, strategies are being developed at the subnational or regional level. All four parts of the United Kingdom have developed their own strategies, and some cantons in Switzerland, autonomous regions of Spain, and *oblasts* in the Russian Federation (such as Tyumen) are developing their own nursing plans. According to replies to a recent WHO global survey *(5)*, the following European countries have developed and adopted plans: the Czech Republic, France, Greece, Hungary, Kazakstan, Latvia, Lithuania, Poland, Sweden, Slovenia, Turkey and the United Kingdom. Furthermore, the Regional Office has noted development activity in this area in Belarus, Belgium, Croatia, Estonia, Finland, Kyrgyzstan, the Netherlands, Romania, Slovakia and Tajikistan, and work beginning in Armenia, Bulgaria, Georgia, the Republic of Moldova, Turkmenistan, Ukraine and Uzbekistan. Some national action plans are the outcome of much debate and are a real tool for future planning, while others are imposed from above, do not attract widespread comment or support, and do not stand much chance of implementation.

Chapter 4 covers in more detail the development and content of a strategic nursing policy. Country-specific situations related to separate milestones, including priority areas for policy and action, are discussed here under the appropriate headings.

LEADERSHIP

Effective leadership is crucial in motivating people, bringing about change, maintaining morale, and establishing the desired role of nurses and nursing services in any health care system. If the profession and individual nurses are to make their full contribution to health care, all policy planning, human resource development and research must involve nurses competent in those areas *(6)*. Nurse leaders must be able to influence decision-making on priority-setting and resource allocation. They need to be respected and accepted as valued contributors, and automatically included in high-level meetings. At the workplace, the nursing voice should be heard in discussions of decisions on direct patient care and on the development and deployment of resources.

Nurses' participation in all aspects of planning at all levels of the health care system is relatively strong in a few countries, such as Iceland, Israel and the United Kingdom. In many others, nurses are not yet seen as a vital part of the policy development group. There is still a long way to go to reach the Vienna vision of nurses "acting as partners in decision-making on the planning and management of local, regional and national health services" *(1)*. Strategies and mechanisms to prepare nurses for their leadership role, and ways to bring about change are discussed extensively in various ICN publications and in *Nursing in action (7)*.

Nursing leadership in Europe is evaluated here by taking a closer look at a few indicators: nurses in government, national nursing associations, international networks, the nurse's role in national policy-making and nurses in management.

Nurses and midwives in government

In 1989, World Health Assembly resolution WHA42.27 urged Member States to "encourage and support the appointment of nursing/midwifery personnel in senior leadership and management positions and to facilitate their participation in planning and implementing the country's health activities" *(8)*. In 1992, resolution WHA45.5 urged Member States to "strengthen managerial and leadership capabilities and reinforce the position of nursing and midwifery personnel in all health care settings" and to "ensure that the contribution of nursing and midwifery is reflected in health policies" *(8)*. The implications of these statements, and some possible ways forward, are explored more fully in Chapter 5.

Having a nursing directorate or unit in the central government, or at least a chief nurse post, is crucial, particularly to develop and implement the national action plan for nursing. Only about a third of European countries have established a specialized nursing (and sometimes midwifery) unit at ministry level. A few countries have a permanent position of chief nurse at the health ministry or its equivalent (see Tables 1 and 2), although doctors hold these posts in some CCEE and NIS. A third of European health ministries have no single permanent position for a nurse, although very few countries have no nurse or midwife employed at the ministry. A few countries, usually those in which nursing education is the sole or main responsibility of the educational sector, have a permanent senior position for a nurse at the education ministry or its equivalent. Despite these still low numbers, there is an encouraging trend. The recent global WHO survey *(5)* revealed that a significant number of countries have increased the number of senior nursing posts at health ministries, or plan to do so. At lower administrative levels, this trend is even clearer. This could mean that nurses' contribution to national policy-making is being recognized in an increasing number of countries; on aggregate more nursing positions exist than in the early 1990s, despite great financial difficulties in health ministries. On the other hand, governments in some countries appear cynically to promise the establishment of leadership posts to nurses and then to do nothing about it. Overall, the visibility of nursing in national governments seems to be rising in all parts of the European Region, albeit slowly.

When a nursing unit or post has been created in government, conditions must be in place for its effective functioning and influence. Reports from all parts of Europe say that, even where health ministries have relatively large nursing departments, nurses must continually fight to make their voices heard. Health ministries alone do not change the world, but the strength of nursing at that level is important in both symbolic and political terms. It is also a fair indicator of the formal power nurses have in a country. The lack of formal power at the top is reflected elsewhere: for example, in the lack of democratic decision-making among members of health care teams in hospitals and communities *(7)*.

As shown in Table 1, most CCEE have now established permanent chief nurse posts at their health ministries or equivalents and most have nurses and/or midwives working at the ministry level. Although the functions and influence vary widely, nearly all chief nurses in the CCEE feel that it is extremely difficult to ensure that nursing issues are taken seriously. In Hungary, the newly enlarged ministerial nursing department has a chief nurse and ten staff, making it the second largest nursing unit at ministry level in Europe. It is responsible for all nursing affairs except university nursing education. Poland has a ministry nursing unit with a chief nurse, a nurse teacher who supervises training schools,

Table 1. Nurses and midwives in central government in the CCEE and NIS

Country	Nursing unit	Midwifery unit	Nursing and midwifery unit	Chief nurse	Chief midwife
Albania					
Armenia				Yes	Yes
Azerbaijan					
Belarus					
Bulgaria			Yes		
Croatia	Yes			Yes	
Czech Republic	Yes	Yes		Yes[a]	Yes[a]
Estonia				Yes	
Georgia				Yes	
Hungary			Yes	Yes	
Kazakstan				Vacant	
Kyrgyzstan			Planned	Yes	
Latvia	Yes			Yes	
Lithuania	Yes			Yes	
Poland			Yes	Yes	
Republic of Moldova				Planned or discussed	
Romania	Yes				
Russian Federation				Planned or discussed	
Slovakia	Yes			Yes	
Slovenia		Yes		Yes	
The Former Yugoslav Republic of Macedonia				Planned or discussed	
Tajikistan				Yes	
Turkmenistan				Yes	
Ukraine				Planned or discussed	
Uzbekistan				Yes	

[a] One person holds both posts.

and a secretary. Here the role of the nursing unit is to advise the deputy minister responsible for nursing, to oversee nursing services, to supervise the education of middle-level staff, and to liaise with the Centre for Postgraduate Medical Education. In Romania, the ministry's deputy director of human resources, a doctor, is responsible for nursing education and leads, with another doctor, a nursing unit of two people.

In the 1980s, all republics in the USSR were instructed to establish chief nurse posts at their health ministries. Many ministries in the NIS therefore still have a chief specialist for nursing or similar post, as in Kyrgyzstan, Latvia and Lithuania, but few other nursing posts. Where they exist, the posts tend to have low status and a doctor usually directs nursing affairs. There are occasional exceptions. The chief nurse in Kyrgyzstan, for example, is well respected and her duties include strategic planning for education, quality assurance and the employment conditions of all middle-level personnel. Georgia, Tajikistan, Turkmenistan and Uzbekistan have recently established chief nurse positions. In Kazakstan the post is frozen, owing to staff cuts in the ministry. In the Republic of Moldova, the Russian Federation and Ukraine, plans are under way to create chief nurse positions, but progress is very slow. These countries have ministry units that deal with nursing education and are staffed by doctors.

Table 2. Nurses in central government in western European countries

Country	Nursing unit	Midwifery unit	Nursing and midwifery unit	Chief nurse	Chief midwife
Austria					
Belgium	Yes			Yes	
Denmark	Yes			Yes	
Finland				Yes	
France				Staff in ministry[a]	Staff in ministry[a]
Germany				In *Länder*	
Greece					
Iceland	Yes		Yes	Focal point for nursing/ midwifery at ministry	
Ireland				Staff in ministry[a]	
Israel			Yes	Yes	
Italy				Staff in ministry[a]	
Luxembourg					
Malta				Yes	
Netherlands	Yes			Yes	
Norway				Staff in ministry[a]	
Portugal					
Spain			Yes	Yes	
Sweden				Yes	
Switzerland	Units or chief nurses/midwives exist at cantonal level				
Turkey	Yes			Yes	
United Kingdom			Yes	Yes	Yes

[a] Nurses and/or midwives work in the health ministry but there is no focal point for nursing.

The position of nurses at the ministry level differs widely in western Europe. Some countries have established posts at the health ministries for chief nurses, who may or may not be supported by nursing (and midwifery) units. The terms of reference of the chief nurses and departments vary, ranging from dealing only with the state hospital nursing services, as in Turkey, to a wide variety of tasks and responsibilities covering areas of nursing legislation, education and practice, as in Israel and the United Kingdom. Other countries comprise a group with separate units at the health ministries, but no chief nurses. Some countries, such as France, Ireland and Norway, have neither chief nurse posts nor nursing departments, but have positions for senior nurses in other departments of the ministry or its equivalent, and have a permanent advisory role to the minister. In Austria, Germany, Italy, Switzerland and elsewhere, the nursing function at the ministry level is weak or absent for various reasons. Nurses are dispersed in different directorates, or nursing is simply not seen as important enough to be represented at the central level.

Role in national policy-making

Active involvement in national decision-making is an essential part of the new role of nurses in the era of health for all. Strong leadership is required at the national level, not only to encourage the development of leaders at other levels but also to emphasize and support the role of nurses in bringing about change *(7)*. The profession has devoted considerable effort to preparing for leadership roles by, for example, identifying and supporting leaders and establishing management development programmes for senior nurses. These take place in all parts of Europe, but in general are more advanced in most countries of western Europe than in the CCEE, and more advanced in the CCEE than in the NIS. In some of these countries, nurses have recently recognized their leadership potential. In others, there is no widespread expression of an urge to participate in national decision- and policy-making, although signs of change are increasing. Inhibiting factors are nurses' and women's lack of formal and informal power in male-dominated, medicalized health care systems. Poor standards of education reinforce this status, which has resulted in low individual and professional self-esteem.

Nurses generally have very restricted opportunities to participate in national decision-making. In some countries, nurses are sometimes elected as members of parliament, as in Finland, Slovenia and the United Kingdom, or appointed or elected to senior political or civil service posts in the health field; for example, the present health minister of Iceland is a nurse. Only a handful of nursing representatives have a permanent position in a national body for health care decision-making, as in Bulgaria, Iceland, Israel and the United Kingdom. Organizations representing nurses have a legal advisory function to these bodies in, for example, Denmark, Italy and the Netherlands. In all the CCEE and NIS, and in the vast majority of western European countries, nurses are not legally entitled to participate in any form of health care decision-making. At best, nurses' representatives are sometimes asked to advise on specific nursing issues. In some countries, nurses are legally responsible for regulating professional matters, such as licensure and professional ethics. This is discussed in the section on regulatory frameworks (pp. 39–50).

In general, the opportunities for nurses to participate in policy-making have increased. There is an encouraging trend in all parts of the Region to involve nurses at least in matters concerning their own profession. Furthermore, nurses are increasingly given legal authority to take part in health care policy-making. The level of involvement, however, varies widely between and within countries. Nurses in the NIS in particular, but also those in most CCEE and some western European countries, still report difficulties in having their voice heard.

In the CCEE, the role of nurses in national policy-making differs between countries. The responsibility of the government chief nurse in Hungary and Slovenia, for example, is to develop clear strategic plans to guide nursing. The role of the chief nurse in Croatia, the Czech Republic, Poland and Slovakia is mainly advisory. NNAs play an active, although usually advisory, role in policy-making related to nursing matters in most countries, such as Bulgaria, Croatia, the Czech Republic, Hungary, Poland, Slovakia and Slovenia. Some of these countries also have national midwifery associations (NMAs). In Poland, the Nurses' and Midwives' Chief Council plays an active role in general health care policy-making, and is involved in planning a new national nursing and midwifery act. In Albania and Romania, policy-making is still not seen as an appropriate role of the nursing profession; neither country has a government chief nurse and the associations are weak, creating a vicious circle that is hard to break.

In all the NIS, nurses make up a large proportion of the health care workforce, but have almost no influence in policy-making or management; a legitimate role here is not acknowledged. There are only a few recognized nurse leaders, and the environment does not favour the development of leadership qualities. Where the role is established, the government chief nurse's part in national policy-making concerning nursing is usually weak. Senior nurses lack professional knowledge and skills in management and leadership, which acts as a barrier to managing changes in the health care system and nursing. The need to improve networking and to develop nursing information systems has been identified as vitally important. Awareness is growing in some countries, such as Estonia, Kyrgyzstan, Latvia, Lithuania and the Republic of Moldova, of the need to develop the legitimate role of nurses in policy-making. The NNAs in the three Baltic states actively try to influence government policy. The President of the Latvian Nursing Association is a member of the body planning the reform of the health care system. The Lithuanian Nursing Association is consulted by the Government, mainly on pay and conditions. In the Republic of Moldova, a Republic Council of Nurses, comprising chief nurses from all over the country, teachers and others, was established in 1993 to develop nursing policy and advise the health ministry. Kazakstan, Kyrgyzstan and Lithuania have also established advisory boards of nurses at the ministry level. The boards' responsibilities include reviewing nursing activities and defining future priorities. In addition, some other countries, such as Estonia, Kazakstan, Kyrgyzstan, Tajikistan, Turkmenistan and Uzbekistan, have also started to use the development of national action plans as a mechanism to bring together a national leadership group, often with the support of WHO.

The role of nurses in national policy-making shows extreme variations in western European countries. In some, such as Iceland, Israel, Spain and the United Kingdom, nurses are actively involved and take a leading role. The CNO, regulatory bodies, professional organizations and trade unions in these countries have a clear role in policy-making at all levels.

The chief nurses of each of the four parts of the United Kingdom (England, Northern Ireland, Scotland and Wales) contribute to health policy. The chief nurse in England is a member of the Policy Board in the Department of Health, and Director of Nursing for the National Health Service (NHS) Executive. The Government appoints the Standing Committee of Nurses and Midwives to advise the Secretary of State for Health, who determines policy on nursing issues. The regulatory bodies established by law, primarily the United Kingdom Central Council for Nursing, Midwifery and Health Visiting, are legally enjoined to protect the public through establishing standards for nursing practice and ensuring the adequate education of practitioners, which inevitably involves these bodies in policy issues. Various professional organizations and trade unions frequently meet the Secretary of State and other officials and thus influence policy-making.

The chief nurse of Israel leads a staff of national supervisors at ministry level whose powers cover the nursing services. They are responsible for hospital, community, mental health, chronic illness and emergency services in their respective divisions. As a group, they formulate nursing policy for Israel and are involved in decision-making at all levels. The nursing unit is currently working on policy determination, a new law on nursing, standards and professional development towards increased clinical specialization.

The situation in most other countries is less favourable: nurses have only an advisory function, carried out by the chief nurse or other senior nurses employed by government, professional associations and/or trade unions. Nurses in many countries (Austria, Belgium, Denmark, Finland, France, Germany, Greece, Ireland, Italy, the Netherlands, Norway, Sweden and Switzerland) report significant difficulties in influencing policy. Sweden, however, established a chief nurse post in 1995. Until recently, nurses in Malta took little part in national policy-making; but a chief nurse post was recently established.

In Finland and France, technical nursing advisers at the health ministry are responsible for advice, representation and assistance. They are linked to regional directorates of health and social affairs by regional nursing advisers and, if necessary, educational advisers. In the Netherlands, the National Centre for Nursing Care is discussing with the Department of Health matters including the effect on nursing of changes in health insurance coverage, demographic changes and the shift from hospital to community care. In addition, the Centre is consulted by the Parliamentary Committee of Public Health, Welfare and Sports. In Italy, the presidents of the national federations of nurses and midwives are members of the two central consultative bodies, the Council for Health Personnel and the National Health Council. In Greece, the Government often consults the Hellenic National Graduate Nurses Association on nursing issues, as well as through informal channels. The National Board for Nursing in Belgium advises the health ministry; it prepares projects and reports on nursing practice and education for discussion and possible formulation as legislation.

Professional associations and trade unions

In many countries the heterogeneity of the roles and tasks associated with nursing, the continuous shifts in the need for nursing and the growth of specialization have resulted in vague definitions of roles and tasks and/or the division of the profession into several – even multiple – groups. This fragmentation is historically and philosophically understandable, and pluralism is always desirable. Nevertheless, countries that have not been able to create some professional unity, perhaps under the aegis of powerful professional associations, seem to have made slower progress in nursing development. Even in the Netherlands, where nursing reaches a high standard, nurses report that the lack of professional unity saps the energy needed for work with other groups. Often in competition or even conflict, various bodies claim to be the voice of nursing in the country. A strong organization with a good working relationship with the chief nurse and other nurses in key positions can assist greatly in monitoring developments and anticipating needs.

With the social changes in the CCEE and NIS, the importance of professional contact and informal peer group support has been more widely recognized. In nearly all the CCEE, nurses have founded or re-established national professional associations, having in most cases recruited 5–10% of the workforce as members to date. Poland's association was originally founded in 1925, and Slovenia's in 1927. The new associations are reaching out internationally to join, or rejoin in some cases, organizations such as ICN and the International Confederation of Midwives (ICM) (see Table 3). At the national level, networks and organizations of nurses, and sometimes other health care professionals, have been established or are well developed. Communication by publications, mail, telephone and fax remains difficult, however, and this restricts opportunities for cooperation in most CCEE.

Trade unions in the CCEE are undergoing a renaissance and many nurses choose to join them as well as or instead of a professional association. Historically, all workers were obliged to join a labour union, while professional associations were mostly frowned on or forbidden. The lack of independence of the old unions has cast a shadow over the new organizations, but they are gradually shaking it off and developing new roles, reinforced by people's growing realization that collective representation and bargaining are even more critical as market forces take hold. Usually the unions focus on pay and conditions, but they are also concerned about equity in health care, education and professional standards. Many trade unions have built international links through affiliation to Public Services International.

In the NIS, the professionalization of nursing is in its infancy. Nurses have founded or re-established independent NNAs or NMAs in only a few countries (see Table 3), and usually the number of members is low. Awareness of the need is growing, however, and nurses have a great desire to act, hampered by lack of resources and expertise, and communication difficulties within and between countries. Estonia, Latvia and Lithuania have relaunched their associations; Estonia's, for example, was first founded in 1923. These associations also come under the umbrella of the Baltic Nurses Association. In Kazakstan and Kyrgyzstan,

Table 3. Professional associations in the CCEE and NIS

Country	Establishment of:		Member of:		
	NNA	NMA	ICN	ICM	Other body[a]
Albania	Yes				
Armenia					
Azerbaijan					
Belarus					
Bulgaria	Yes	Yes	Yes		
Croatia	Yes		Applied		
Czech Republic	Yes	Yes	Applied	Yes	1
Estonia	Yes		Yes		2
Georgia	In progress				
Hungary	Yes[b]		Yes		1
Kazakstan	In progress[c]				
Kyrgyzstan	In progress				
Latvia	Yes	Yes	Yes		2
Lithuania	Yes				2
Poland	Yes		Yes		1
Republic of Moldova	Yes[c]				
Romania	Yes	Yes	Applied		
Russian Federation	No[c]				
Slovakia	Yes		Applied		
Slovenia	Yes		Yes		
The Former Yugoslav Republic of Macedonia	Yes				
Tajikistan	In progress				
Turkmenistan	In progress				
Ukraine	In progress[c]				
Uzbekistan					

[a] 1 = Workgroup of European Nurse Researchers; 2 = Baltic Nurses Association.
[b] The Hungarian Nurses Association has a separate midwifery section.
[c] Organizations exist at the subnational and regional levels.

NNAs are planned, and one was founded in the Republic of Moldova after the first-ever national meeting of 250 nurses in May 1994: a remarkable achievement based not on money but on determination, networking and grass-roots activity. In the Russian Federation, the role of professional organizations is not clearly established, but some internal networks exist, built on leading institutions such as the Faculty of Nursing at the I.M. Sechenov Moscow Medical Academy (now a WHO collaborating centre for nursing) and the Central Institute for Advanced

Table 4. Professional associations in western Europe

Country	Establishment of:		Member of:		
	NNA	NMA	ICN	ICM	Other body[a]
Austria	Yes	Yes	Yes	Yes	1, 4, 5
Belgium	Yes	Yes	Yes	Yes	1, 2, 5
Denmark	Yes	Yes	Yes	Yes	2–5
Finland	Yes	Yes	Yes	Yes	2–5
France	Yes	Yes	Yes		1, 2, 4, 5
Germany	Yes	Yes	Yes	Yes	2, 4, 5
Greece	Yes	Yes	Yes	Yes	1, 2, 4, 5
Iceland	Yes	Yes	Yes	Yes	2, 3, 5
Ireland	Yes		Yes	Yes	2, 4
Israel	Yes	Yes	Yes	Yes	5
Italy	Yes	Yes	Yes	Yes	1, 2, 4, 5
Luxembourg	Yes	Yes	Yes	Yes	1, 2, 4, 5
Malta	Yes	Yes	Yes	Yes	
Netherlands	Yes	Yes	Yes	Yes	2, 4, 5
Norway	Yes	Yes	Yes	Yes	2, 3, 5
Portugal	Yes	Yes	Yes		1, 4
Spain	Yes	Yes	Yes	Yes	1, 2, 4, 5
Sweden	Yes	Yes	Yes	Yes	2–5
Switzerland	Yes	Yes	Yes	Yes	1, 2, 5
Turkey	Yes		Yes		
United Kingdom	Yes	Yes	Yes	Yes	2, 4, 5

[a] 1 = European Nursing Group; 2 = European Nursing Quality Network; 3 = Northern Nurses Federation; 4 = Standing Committee of Nurses of the European Community; and 5 = The Workgroup of European Nurse Researchers.

Medical Studies (CIAMS) in Moscow. Some attempts are being made to establish local and regional professional associations. For example, a Moscow Nurses Association has been formed and is receiving help from European associations, and there are others in regional centres such as Mari and Samara. Local associations have also been formed in Almaty, Kazakstan and Kiev, Ukraine. This regional or local development is probably more likely to succeed, and to spread through a ripple effect, than attempts to found organizations at the national level in the absence of resources and infrastructures. It is also more realistic in very large countries such as Kazakstan and the Russian Federation.

All countries in western Europe have nursing associations (see Table 4), ranging from single organizations in Iceland, Malta and Norway to over 50 separate organizations in France and the Netherlands. Except in Spain, membership is voluntary. In all countries except Belgium and the Netherlands, the total membership exceeds 80% of nurses. Accurate figures are not always easy to obtain or verify, however, and many people have duplicate membership. Nurses and midwives are often members of trade unions for health care professionals or civil servants or those specifically for nurses and/or midwives.

Almost all countries, except Turkey, have one or more separate midwifery associations. An exception is Ireland, where midwives are members of the Irish Nurses Organization and the midwives' section of the National Council of Nurses. The proportion of midwives belonging to a midwifery organization usually exceeds 90%.

Networks

European nurses should share knowledge and learn from each other's problems and successes by "setting up information systems and increasing communication and the dissemination of information and research results through national, regional and international networks" *(1)*. Cooperation is needed within national networks of nurses and midwives to steer professional development at all levels, as is cooperation at the international level with ICN, ICM, Public Services International (PSI), the Standing Committee of Nurses of the European Union (PCN), and the Workgroup of European Nurse Researchers (WENR), and between midwives in ICM and the EU Midwives' Liaison Group. Important newer networks include the Leaders in Nursing Network (LINK) convened by WHO, which comprises anglophone and russophone groups in which chief nurses or the nearest equivalent from nearly all European countries (including all the CCEE and NIS) are represented. The Regional Office also established a European network of WHO collaborating centres for nursing and midwifery to reinforce the work of a similar global network. Many different networks and associations bring together nurses and midwives interested in a particular clinical specialty or other field. Until recently, they catered almost exclusively to western Europe, but membership is gradually spreading further afield through such organizations as the European Nursing Quality Network (EUROQUAN).

While the range and variety of networks are welcome, they are in danger of echoing the fragmentation often seen at the national level. Further action is being debated on how to bring the networks closer together through, for example, an ad hoc European nursing forum or some other, more formal group.

Role in management

Nurses have been managing the delivery of patient care for many years. Organizations such as ICN, ILO and WHO have stressed the need for nurses to be partners in the planning and management of health services and to manage nursing autonomously. Many nurses are effective managers, but the management function in nursing often goes unrecognized and unrewarded. Despite having heavy management responsibilities, senior nurses may remain without influence on planning and budget allocation. Apparent seniority in the health service hierarchy may not be reflected in input to decision-making. This is true in many countries but especially in the CCEE and NIS; the autonomy and influence that nurses enjoy when managing nursing are closely linked to nursing's relationship with other disciplines and its status. In many countries, nurses are expected to carry out a housekeeping role that may be reflected in the tasks of the nurse manager.

Female nurses experience particular difficulty in asserting a right to take part in decision-making, partly because this is nearly always dominated by male doctors and/or career administrators who naturally assume leadership. Furthermore, socialization as a woman and a nurse may teach subordination and passivity. (Men in nursing have been conspicuously more successful than women in reaching senior positions, often by dint of presenting themselves as managers rather than as nurses.) Nurses are therefore easily marginalized in the management culture, particularly if their role is unacknowledged. This in turn renders them less effective. Nevertheless, skilled nurses are needed to manage not only nurses but also the standards, organization and delivery of nursing. This presupposes strong educational programmes in which they can learn to blend nursing and management skills.

The nurse's role in management varies significantly in the CCEE. In Croatia, the Czech Republic, Hungary, Poland, Slovakia and Slovenia, nurses are recognized as important members of the multidisciplinary PHC team, and are involved in planning care at the local and district levels. In the clinical setting, nurses manage nurses, and the responsibility for the quality of nursing rests with senior nurses. In Romania, there are plans to have a chief nurse in every hospital with more than 300 beds, although the position will not be one of high status, without real involvement in decision-making or independent control of the nursing workforce or budget. Most CCEE have a director of nursing services in each hospital, accountable to the hospital administrator, and a head nurse in each department and ward. Elsewhere, nurses are more or less subordinate to medical authority. The typical chief nurse of a hospital is mainly expected to advise the hospital administrator or medical director on nursing matters, rather than to take the lead in nursing matters. In all countries, head nurses manage nursing at the ward and department levels. Nurse managers now have increasing opportunities for training in many of the CCEE.

According to the old Soviet legislation, each health care facility in the NIS should have a chief nurse to assist the chief doctor or hospital director. (Although the NIS are gradually reviewing and replacing the old legislation, the model is still influential.) A feldsher may occupy the post, but all candidates must have five years' experience and have completed a management course. In theory, the chief nurse is elected by a council of nurses in each hospital; each establishment with more than 15 nurses must have a council that discusses nursing topics and elects nurse leaders. The senior nurse in each department or ward reports to the doctor in charge and organizes all nursing activities.

Nearly all the NIS show growing awareness of the need for change, and more demands for autonomy and recognition for nursing. Many have chief nurses at the *oblast* or district level, who may be responsible for organizing continuing education as well as supervising nursing services. In Uzbekistan, for example, chief nurse posts have been introduced in municipal and district health departments whose responsibilities include registering middle-level personnel, supervising the upgrading of qualifications, and organizing continuing education. In Kazakstan, the post of chief nurse on the Almaty City Health Board was established in 1989 to lead the city's 10 700 nursing staff. She works with a team of nurses but lacks management training, and says her major problem is acceptance by other professionals. This is an essential point; in the NIS, the nurse has little or no role as a partner in planning and management of health services at the lower or intermediate administrative levels.

In most western European countries, nursing and nurses are managed by nurses who have completed postbasic courses in management and/or clinical specialties. (The exceptions are Malta, Sweden and Turkey, where nurses in clinical settings are still subordinate to doctors, to whom they must report on patient care.) The director of nursing is responsible for managing, coordinating and assessing nursing services, usually working as part of a hospital or PHC management team consisting of a doctor, a nurse and an administrator, but sometimes directly responsible to the chief executive or administrator. The nursing director often has much independence in leadership and the deployment of human resources: assessing workloads, monitoring quality and organizing continuing education. Nurse managers usually take part in planning as members of a multidisciplinary team. In some countries, however, the autonomy and status of nurse managers have suffered from the introduction of general management principles and practices, with a concomitant downgrading of professional influence. (Doctors also complain of this.) The wholesale introduction of general management in the British NHS in the 1980s, for example, resulted in many nurse management posts being cut and other staff taking responsibility for nursing management functions traditionally carried out by nurses. Senior nurses who aspire to management positions have been obliged to play down their nursing background and skills.

Regulatory Frameworks

WHO and its Member States advocate the use of PHC to achieve health for all. This commitment is set out in the Declaration of Alma-Ata *(9)*. At the 1988 European Conference on Nursing in Vienna *(1)*, the nurses of Europe expressed their own commitment and the support it required:

> 1. All nurses, their professional associations, nongovernmental organizations and volunteer groups should be strong advocates for policies and programmes for health for all at national, regional and local levels.
>
> 2. Innovative nursing services should be developed that focus on health rather than disease; patterns of work should be appropriate, efficient and conducive to primary health care. Governments, health authorities and nurses' professional organizations should take urgent steps to remove factors that inhibit this process and should draw up or modify legislation and regulation to ensure that nurses are able to meet their responsibilities as front-line workers in primary health care.

Regulation and legislation may sound somewhat academic and removed from practice, but they play a major part, for good or ill, in determining the scope and quality of nursing throughout the European Region.

Legislation and regulations

All European countries have legislation to determine the practice of the health professions. In addition, other control mechanisms may have a bearing on nursing practice, such as laws regulating the professions of medicine and pharmacy, rules and regulations of a statutory nursing board or council, regulations of the health ministry, professional codes related to standards and ethics, and even the rules or by-laws of an individual institution *(10)*. Legislative and regulatory practices and mechanisms vary between countries and within them, where regulation is the responsibility of a state or province, as in Belgium, Germany and Switzerland.

Nursing legislation in countries such as Norway sets out detailed requirements for mandatory licensure for practice. The laws of other countries, such as the Netherlands, allow nursing to be practised by unlicensed persons, but prohibit the use of the designation "nurse" except by duly qualified people. These laws typically define practice in broad and often vague terms. A 1986 ICN report on the regulation of nurses *(11)* concluded that:

- nursing enjoyed no universal definition of function and no universal standards of education and practice;
- the scope of nursing practice as defined by law was often more restrictive than nurses' abilities and the public need for their services; and
- education standards in statutory regulation were generally inadequate to fulfil the nursing role in PHC.

The report noted variations in the role of NNAs in setting standards for the profession and its members; this role was weak in some countries, and clear and powerful in others. Despite improvements all over Europe, these statements remain largely valid.

The underlying principles of and rationale for the regulation of professional practice are of universal application. ICN and WHO *(10)* agree that a nursing regulatory system should:

- establish, monitor and enforce essential standards; improve and sustain education, training and practice; and provide a framework for nursing practice relevant to meeting the health needs of the population and protecting the public;
- provide public authority, credibility, protection and support to permit nurses to reach the maximum extent of their capabilities;
- promote regulation of the nursing profession by nurses to ensure appropriate standards of education and practice;
- encourage nurses to participate in and influence public debate on health policy; and
- ensure that each practitioner is accountable to the public for nursing practice.

Legal and regulatory frameworks to govern the profession should be complemented by provisions in labour regulations to guarantee and safeguard practitioners' working conditions and remuneration. These aspects of professional life are of central importance to the role of nurses, and need to be considered in relation to improving health services. The member states of ILO have repeatedly recommended such provisions for nurses; their content and importance are extensively discussed below (pp. 81–91).

WHO has formulated a flexible model for nursing regulatory mechanisms, stemming from legislation *(10)*. It includes three kinds of mechanism, each of which affects the others: primary legislation, rules and regulations, and codes and guidelines.

Primary legislation is an act of the legislature establishing a regulatory body and defining its formation, composition and principal functions. It addresses powers to make rules and to give advice or set guidelines on admission to, and the content of, educational programmes; to approve educational programmes, examinations and assessments; to grant licensure and maintain a register of qualified nurses; to regulate entry to the register and removal from the register for professional misconduct or other reasons; and entitlement to the use of the title nurse.

Rules or regulations have the power of law and provide:

- mechanisms for licensure or the establishment of a register, addressing:
  - entry to and removal from the register;
  - criteria for registration of overseas applicants;
  - registration renewal from time to time;
- rules on training, addressing:
  - its type and standard;
  - length;
  - education and other admission requirements;
  - competences or outcomes;
  - examinations;
  - approval of training schools or colleges; and
- rules on practice, if they are seen as appropriate.

Codes may be established on ethics, practice or conduct, and guidelines may arise from and detail the clauses of codes. Examples include guidelines on advertising nursing services, confidentiality and the administration of drugs. In addition, circulars, possibly issued at regular intervals, may give advice on all aspects of concern to the regulatory body and the response of the profession in relation to them *(10)*.

Regulatory frameworks that govern nursing practice may be established by law in different ways: through statutory regulations, custom, convention or consensus. In essence, nursing regulation means bringing the practice of nurses and the preparation of practitioners under statutory control, and giving the designated authority the right and power to check, verify and determine limits and to take steps to keep practice within these limits.

Regulations with implications for nursing have been issued by both the European Community (EC) and the Council of Europe (CE) as directives or recommendations, respectively, for their member states. Since 1994, the EC guidelines have also been in force in the countries belonging to the European Free Trade Association (EFTA), except Switzerland. Some of the crucial regulations deal with issues of mutual recognition of diplomas and the quality of education and include:

- the 1967 CE recommendations on nursing education;
- the 1977 EC directive on mutual recognition of general nurse diplomas and the establishment of general nurses in other member states (77/452/EEC);
- the 1977 EC directive on the skills required of general nurses, to be obtained through a general (primary and secondary) education of at least 10 years' duration and a full-time training of three years, covering at least 4600 hours of theoretical and practical instruction, plus an important annex on the theoretical and clinical–practical elements to be incorporated into the education of general nurses (77/453/EEC);
- the 1989 directive (89/595/EEC) amending directives 77/452/EEC and 77/453/EEC.

The 1977 EC directives have been very influential not only within the EU but also in countries outside it, including the CCEE and NIS *(12)*. The directives have informally acquired the status of international standards, although they deal explicitly with the mobility of the workforce and the harmonization of qualifications between countries, and were not explicitly formulated to set or raise standards. Nearly 20 years on, some countries have not implemented them, although all EU and EFTA members except the United Kingdom have now legally recognized overseas nursing diplomas as defined by them.

Important CE recommendations include that made in 1983 on post-basic education (further training), particularly in clinical nursing specialization, nursing education, and nursing management and administration, and those made in 1995 on nursing research. In addition, the CE health committee has accepted a recent report of a CE working party on the role and education of nurses, and the European Commission is due to consider the report in the light of its existing directives related to nursing education.

In the 1980s and early 1990s, there was much debate on the implementation of a directive on the mutual recognition of qualifications other than those of the nurse responsible for general care, especially in the fields of paediatric and psychiatric nursing. In 1992 a directive on specialists was prepared by the Advisory Committee on Training of Nurses (ACTN), but difficulties in implementation have arisen as a result of:

- problems in countries' recognition of specialist diplomas for which they do not have equivalents;
- the danger of setting only minimum requirements, which may dilute the high standards fought for and achieved in some countries; and
- the whole question of specialist training, as there is an increasing tendency throughout the world for nurses to be trained as generalists.

A 1992 WHO survey of health ministries revealed that nursing and midwifery legislation still restricted practice at the national level, and led to the underuse of the abilities of nurses and midwives in many countries, especially the CCEE and NIS. At the same time, nurses and midwives in some countries were performing duties not covered by law, thereby jeopardizing their personal and professional standing. The 1992 World Health Assembly resolution urged Member States to enact legislation or take appropriate measures to ensure good nursing and midwifery services *(8)*. In the 1990s, many countries in the European Region have enacted or begun to review legislation aimed at protecting the public through high-quality nursing and/or midwifery education and services. The CCEE and NIS that are in the process of changing their nursing education systems, such as the Czech Republic, Estonia, Hungary, Latvia, Lithuania, Romania and Slovenia, take account of the EC directives.

Almost all European countries have made, are making or are planning changes in legislation on:

- training and education requirements;
- the introduction of equal opportunity policies;
- new standards of practice for maternity care and other nursing specialties (as in Norway, Sweden and the United Kingdom);
- new policies on the utilization of nursing personnel (as in Germany, Italy and Slovenia);
- the codification of ethical principles for nurses and the role of the nurse (as in France and Lithuania); and

- the review and updating of regulations governing nursing and midwifery practice, including licensing (as in Estonia, Germany, Hungary, Poland and Norway).

Some countries pointed to a need for a new regulatory system for the profession and/or institutions employing nurses (as in France, the Netherlands and Slovakia). There is a welcome tendency to make nursing legislation more flexible by describing the roles, functions and competences of the nurse, as opposed to listing the clinical tasks to be performed.

As a consequence of recent social and political reforms, most of the CCEE have improved the legislative position of all health care workers, including nurses. Many have implemented a new law on health care and/or health insurance that recognizes nurses as professional health workers. In Croatia, the Czech Republic, Hungary and Slovakia, the profession has received more authority over nursing practice in different settings and education, but legislation on nursing practice remains very restrictive in Albania, Bulgaria, Poland and Romania. Most CCEE are particularly active in establishing a new legal basis for nurse education and a system of professional registration. A new phenomenon in some, such as the Czech Republic, Hungary, Slovakia and Slovenia, is the legal possibility for nurses to be independent private practitioners. Good examples of countries' activities to review their legislation and bring it more into line with their new circumstances come from the former Czechoslovakia, which passed several laws concerning nursing in 1991/1992:

- an education law, bringing education into line with European standards for nursing education;
- a law on care provision, allowing private practice;
- a law on general health insurance, allowing direct payment to workers for services;
- a decree detailing the extended role of nurses in PHC and home nursing;
- a law on wages, ensuring adequate wages for nursing staff;
- a law on people's health, enabling midwives to work independently;
- a law on health workers, creating a new type of educational programme for midwives; and
- a law on health care provision in non-state health facilities, establishing role boundaries and regulating the independent work of the midwife.

Almost all the NIS are updating their legislation. They inherited the old public health law of the USSR, which dealt with all categories of health worker – doctors, pharmacists, nurses, feldshers, midwives and laboratory technicians. It defined them as people who had obtained the necessary qualifications to practise their profession, after having completed appropriate studies and passed a prescribed examination. This law severely restricted nursing practice by setting out a limited list of mostly clinical tasks:

- caring for patients, including care of the body, diet, bedding and assistance in emergencies;
- observation of weight, pulse, temperature, respiration, skin colour, excretion and psychological condition;
- carrying out medical instructions regarding drugs, intramuscular or subcutaneous injections, lavage, probing, pre-operative preparation, monitoring of anaesthesia, dressings, and assistance in therapeutic and diagnostic activities;
- collaboration in pre- and post-therapeutic intervention;
- health education; and
- maintenance of medical and technical equipment.

In Estonia, Kyrgyzstan, Lithuania and the Russian Federation, governments have started reforming legislation on health care and health care professionals. The Russian Federation adopted a new public health law at the end of 1993. It deals with all categories of health workers, but still restricts nursing practice, and new legislation is being discussed. Lithuania adopted a new national health care law in 1994 that gives nurses a new status as independent professionals, and further legislation on nursing practice is being prepared; the Committee of Standards sets norms for nursing assistants and ethical principles for nurses. In Kyrgyzstan, attempts at reform have begun and new legislation was issued in 1991. Estonia established a licensing system for nurses, although the health organization law of 1994 did not include a new status for nursing.

All countries of western Europe have legislation on nursing practice and education, but its scope and content vary widely. In some, legislation on nursing practice is part of the overall law on health care personnel (as in the Netherlands) and/or hospital practice (as in Belgium). Most countries (such as France, Italy, the United Kingdom and the Nordic countries) have incorporated specific regulations for nurses' responsibilities, competences and duties in laws on nursing acts or their equivalents. In almost all countries except Switzerland, the title nurse is legally protected. Countries such as Austria are strengthening central legislation and/or regulation of nursing practice while others, such as the Netherlands, are reducing the role of the central government. Several countries (such as Israel, Malta and Turkey) are planning new legislation on nursing practice.

Some examples show the large differences among western European countries in the content of legislation and the role of government in regulating nursing practice. All parts of the United Kingdom have implemented an act on nurses, midwives and health visitors. The professions have considerable authority in formulating, setting standards for and evaluating practice and education; it is vested primarily in a statutory regulatory body, the United Kingdom Central Council for Nursing, Midwifery and Health Visiting, whose mandate is not to advance the professions but to safeguard the public. In France, a 1991 law aims at reforming hospital services, including the establishment of nursing services in hospitals directed by a head nurse, and stipulates their composition, designation and functioning; 80% of establishments have introduced these reforms. A 1993 government decree defines the role and professional acts of nurses; it accentuates the nurse's participation in continuing education, disease prevention and health education, and role in primary and community care. In Spain, nursing staff in the public sector are covered by the statute on non-doctor health staff in social security institutions, which deals with circumstances relating to service provision, such as the functions of nursing staff, their rights and obligations, a disciplinary code and a system of access to posts. Nursing staff working in other institutions, such as those of provincial authorities, the Red Cross and private enterprises, are regulated by the labour regulations for health workers through collective bargaining agreements.

Registration and licence to practise

Registration is the process through which people are assessed and given status on a register attesting to their ability or qualifications. Registration usually entitles a person to bear a specific title. Although registration in nursing limits the use of a particular title to registered nurses, it does not usually limit practice to them, and is therefore usually called voluntary or permissive regulation. Licensure, on the other hand, is a more powerful mechanism – a mandatory or compulsory process that restricts practice to licensed individuals, and permits people with predetermined minimal competences to practise nursing *(7)*. ILO recognized the importance of having a system regulating requirements for entrance into nursing practice in Article 4 of its 1977 Convention on nursing *(4)*: "National laws or regulations shall specify the requirements for the practice of nursing and limit that practice to persons who meet these requirements".

Registration and licensure systems in the CCEE adopt different approaches and are at different stages of development. Croatia, the Czech Republic, Hungary, Poland, Slovakia and Slovenia have established systems mainly involving the registration of certificates. For example, in Hungary the Central Training Institute for Qualified Nurses maintains records of all nursing certificates, including those of auxiliaries, while the Institute of Public Health performs this task in Slovenia. A register of practising nurses is usually maintained at a lower administrative level. In Slovenia, professional registration is part of the responsibilities of the district nursing chambers, while in Poland registration is decentralized to the 49 voivodships or regions. The nurse or midwife is obliged to register with the registration department of the nurses' and midwives' district council of the voivodship before practising, and to inform the registration unit whenever changing place of work. The licence to practise can be given for a limited or unlimited period. Health professionals are fully accountable for their work and those who violate the principles of ethics, dignity and professional scrupulousness are subject to penalties that include reprimand, censure, payment of a fine and removal of the right to practise for a limited or unlimited period. These matters are determined by the Regional Professional Supervision Commission at voivodship level, and the Professional Supervision Appeal Commission at the health ministry.

Albania, Bulgaria and Romania have no national registration systems. The development of such a system is a priority in Bulgaria, and has been identified as important by the Romanian Nurses Association. Central authorities that do not recognize the role of nurses and midwives as autonomous professionals do not, however, devote their attention to establishing such systems.

Professional licensure is almost nonexistent in the CCEE. The exceptions are the countries that have recently introduced private practice: Croatia, the Czech Republic, Hungary, Slovakia and Slovenia. A licence to practise privately usually needs to be obtained from the health ministry or its equivalent. In all other cases, a licence to practise is automatically granted after the successful completion of training. Nevertheless, completion of training is not a requirement to perform nursing duties, as shown by the high numbers of unqualified nursing assistants in almost all CCEE. Few of the CCEE yet comply with Article 4 of the ILO Convention.

In most NIS except Estonia and the Russian Federation, there is no system of professional registration or licensure, and no country complies with the ILO Convention. The Russian Federation has a state system of qualification verification that consists of an oral examination. People who pass the examination receive a higher grade and a salary increase. A licence is obligatory for private practice. Estonia has a system of diploma registration, in which all graduate nurses are registered with the education ministry. The central registration of practising nurses is planned. Kyrgyzstan is attempting to establish a system based on the registration of certificates. A ministerial decree of August 1991 outlines the licensing of middle-level health personnel: a positive move towards establishing a full professional registration system.

Most western European countries have a national registration or licensure system, mainly based on certificates of qualification. The register is usually held centrally by the health ministry, the education ministry or a legally designated national body, although the validation of the title is sometimes decentralized to lower administrative levels. Exceptions include Norway, where nurse practitioners must have one year of postbasic experience before registration. In Austria, Belgium and Germany, registration has been totally decentralized to the regional level, while Turkey has no registration system. Diplomas awarded in Switzerland are registered with the Swiss Red Cross, and some specialties are registered by the Swiss Nursing Association. The Association has petitioned the Government for the recognition of certificates of competence, diplomas and postbasic qualifications by a national authority, and for the protection of the corresponding nursing titles at the national level. In most other countries, except Turkey, the title nurse and the practice of nursing are restricted to people who hold an official diploma in nursing, thus complying with the ILO Convention. In the Netherlands, as a consequence of the law on professions in health care, all nurses must re-register before 1 December 1997 to keep their title. By means of this law, the Dutch Government has introduced the more powerful mechanism of licensure, with the introduction of a set of acts specifically reserved to nurses. Belgium, through a 1974 law, also has some reserved acts, and an unqualified person in Denmark can risk legal measures if she or he claims to another lay person to be a nurse *(12)*.

The registration of postbasic specialties is normally a task of the profession itself, usually of the professional associations. In some countries this is carried out centrally by the health ministry or a designated national body, as is the case in Israel. In addition, most countries maintain registers of practising nurses, usually at lower administrative levels. The profession itself is responsible for registration, however, in Ireland, Italy, Spain and the United Kingdom. Payment of a registration fee is not unusual. For example, nurses in the United Kingdom pay an initial fee and further fees every three years; those in Ireland pay an annual fee.

Besides registration, nursing councils are usually responsible for the monitoring of professional discipline. In all countries, official registration and/or licence to practise can be withdrawn if the person is proved unworthy. Such a decision is usually made by the authorities responsible for registration or licensure. A private nurse practitioner normally needs an additional licence to practise, obtained from the district or regional health authorities.

Self-regulation

In addition to statutory regulation, authorities within the profession may regulate nurses and nursing, as shown above. This professional self-regulation occurs at several levels: the individual practitioner, the workplace team, the health care or academic institution, the professional association or trade union, and the ICN and ICM *(13)*. While the goal of external regulation is to protect the public, self-regulation goes beyond that. It mainly aims at improving the quality of services while protecting the public and stimulating the advancement of the profession. Self-regulation includes setting standards and codes and keeping nurses' knowledge and skills up to date.

In countries where professional organizations work hand in hand with the government (for example, when NNAs and NMAs are created by statute or have statutory authority for registration and/or licensing), it is usually clear who speaks for nursing and midwifery in the regulatory process. Sometimes, however, there is ambiguity or conflict, particularly about the authority of the government, professions and associations and trade unions. Confusion and competition are growing with the proliferation of nursing specialties and special interest groups, some of whom are independent of the associations. Where the profession does not have the apparatus for developing a unanimous position, or where opinion varies widely, each interest group seeks representation and coalition with compatible interests in the process of governing, and the profession as a whole is not represented in the process.

In the spirit of health for all, WHO advocates pluralism and participation in the policy process, rather than favouring one form of authority over another (see Chapter 4). ICN also attempts to separate governmental and professional responsibility, stressing a joint effort *(14)*: "Distinction needs to be made between the right to practise, which is a provision of law, and the standards for practice, which must be determined by the profession". These assumptions imply the responsibility of the government and the profession to work jointly towards controlling licensure. For example, legislation may limit licensure to people whose practice conforms to acceptable standards, and may withdraw it from those whose malpractice or other unsatisfactory behaviour or conduct calls for disciplinary action. Nevertheless, the profession is responsible for preparing its own code of ethics and establishing standards for practice *(14)*.

Ethical standards and good professional conduct are extremely important issues, and some regulatory bodies, professional associations and trade unions have addressed them by drawing up codes of conduct or position statements. In 1973, ICN developed a code for nurses, used widely by NNAs, addressing ethical concepts and standards of conduct for the profession worldwide *(15,16)*. Because a single code cannot be applied to all societies, there is a need to adapt it to each country's circumstances, as the NNAs of Denmark, Ireland, Norway, Poland, Spain and the United Kingdom have done.

The Role of the Nurse

WHO has defined the mission of nursing in society as helping individuals, families and groups to determine and achieve their physical, mental and social potential, within the environments in which they live and work. This requires nurses to develop and perform functions that prevent ill health and promote and maintain good health. Nursing also includes the planning and delivery of care during illness and rehabilitation, and encompasses the physical, mental and social aspects of life as they affect health, illness, disability and dying. Nurses ensure the active involvement of the individual and his or her family, friends, social group and community, as appropriate, in all aspects of health care, thus encouraging self-reliance and self-determination. Nurses also work as partners with members of other professions and occupations involved in providing health and related services *(7)*.

The functions of the nurse derive directly from the mission of nursing in society *(7)*. These functions remain constant, regardless of the place and time in which nursing care is given, the health status of the individual or group to be served, or the resources available. Furthermore, the functions should be reflected in the legislation governing nursing in each country. In the light of nursing's mission in society, nurses' role should focus on:

- promoting and maintaining health and preventing disease;
- involving individuals, their families and communities in care and enabling them to take responsibility for their health;

- working to reduce inequities in access to health care services and to satisfy the needs of the whole population, especially the underserved;
- taking part in multidisciplinary and multisectoral collaboration;
- ensuring the quality of care and appropriate use of technology; and
- restructuring, reorienting and strengthening basic programmes of nursing education to enable nurses to carry out their functions in both hospital and community.

Developing a shared vision of the ideal role of nursing in society has been discussed at many meetings of nursing leaders in the European Region (see Annexes 1–4). The 1988 Vienna Declaration *(1)* urged nurses to develop their role by:

> acting as partners in decision-making in the planning and management of local, regional and national health services, playing a greater role in empowering individuals, families and communities to become more self-reliant and to take charge of their health development, and providing clear and valid information on the favourable and adverse consequences of various types of behaviour, and on the merits and costs of different options for care.

Continuing discussions after 1988, involving nursing leaders throughout the Region, including new Member States, reaffirmed the relevance of the Declaration and the accompanying Conference recommendations, concluding that they continued to provide a vision to guide the Region's nurses and midwives *(17)*. New attitudes and values need to be fostered among all health professionals, citizens and related groups that are consistent with the European policy for health for all *(18)* and the PHC approach *(9)*. Nursing can best fulfil its potential in PHC and hospital settings when education provides a sound foundation for practice, especially in the community, and when nurses take account of the social aspects of health needs and have a broad understanding of health development. Policies should be adopted and activities identified to enable nurses to practise with sufficient autonomy to carry out their new role.

Such statements, and similar ones from around the world, are often made, but there are widely contrasting perceptions of the demands and expectations placed on nurses, and of nursing's social and professional status. Since the beginning of the 1980s, the increases in people's expectations and expressed needs have led to a stronger demand for skilled nursing. Nurses are increasingly perceived as having not only the traditional professional (or perhaps womanly) attributes of discretion, readiness to serve, dedication and altruism, but also intellectual qualities and expertise evidenced by competence and technical and psychosocial ability and skills. Thus, the role of the nurse has expanded considerably, but nurses' demands show that they still believe their social and professional status is too low. Their demands particularly address the following factors:

- the increasing diversity and complexity and evolving character of nursing work, which has many different aspects (technical, intellectual, relational and educational);
- the radical changes taking place in nursing work, resulting from advances in medical technology (which necessitate new specialist skills to deal not only with technology but also the human consequences of saving or prolonging life) and from the development of new, more sophisticated concepts of care;
- the nature of professional practice, which demands competence and the acceptance of individual responsibility and accountability *(19)*;
- the need for higher qualifications, which has resulted from demographic and epidemiological change and professional and social pressure.

Entry requirements are stricter, courses are much more demanding, and today's nurse is often educated to the level of a university degree and beyond.

Real and lasting changes in health care require that health professionals and patients or clients take on different roles and functions. This cannot be accomplished solely by changes in financing and/or delivery structures. Cultural factors and formal and informal interpersonal relationships – including the role of the professions in health care and society – must be taken into account. The definition of new nursing roles and functions should have effects extending beyond the profession: the establishment of a dialogue between all interest groups – based on more equal relationships, trust and willingness to talk, listen and change – is a first and important step and outcome of the reform process.

The distance between the visions of nursing leaders and actual practice is most clearly visible in the CCEE and NIS, where the role of the nurse is legally restricted to a prescribed number of tasks, in effect limiting it to that of a doctor's assistant. The word for nurse in the Russian language, which has colonized the evolution of professional terminology in many CCEE and NIS, literally means a medical sister or brother or middle-level medical worker. In most of these countries, nurses still work on the instructions of doctors, providing a service to other professionals rather than to patients. This makes nursing dependent on and subordinate to medicine, which creates major problems for the development of the profession. Most doctors and, indeed, many nurses believe this professional hierarchy is necessary and proper. Very few have had the chance to see the modern western European nurse in action, so they lack the knowledge to assess the validity of their current situation.

In the CCEE and NIS, nurses work in a variety of settings including hospitals, polyclinics, rural health centres, maternity homes, children's homes, factories and kindergartens. Because of their low status and education and the oversupply of doctors in most countries, doctors often carry out nursing work and nurses mostly do the work of assistants – tasks that in western European countries would be carried out by support workers with minimal or no qualifications. The NIS nurse is usually found cleaning equipment and floors, preparing meals, performing secretarial and other paper work, making observations, giving treatments and performing specific tasks on doctors' orders; she or he gives little direct patient care, apart from some tending tasks, and no psychosocial care. In some places, independent decision-making on the planning and implementation of nursing care is nil, medical domination total and nursing autonomy nonexistent.

The case is rather different with another group of middle-level staff in the NIS: the feldshers. Although they are sometimes called doctors' assistants, they have a more independent role, especially in rural areas, and may admit and examine patients, prescribe care, treatment and drugs, perform minor surgery and make home visits. This role is discussed more fully below, and needs further investigation.

Nurses, midwives and feldshers in the CCEE and NIS are mainly women and they often receive no recognition as professionals from the community or the medical profession. This is reflected in their low salaries, often comparable to those of unskilled labourers. Facile comparisons with western countries should be avoided, however, as doctors in the CCEE and NIS also have relatively low status and salaries, and the division of labour is not a simple matter of professional recognition. In general, nurses' status, recognition and professional autonomy are greater in the CCEE than in the NIS, and are developing faster for many reasons, including the better economic situation, greater donor assistance, different cultural and social assumptions about women, and proximity to western countries.

The position of nurses in some of the CCEE, such as Albania, Bulgaria and Romania, is not much better than in the NIS, however. In

Poland, the role of the nurse is determined by the doctor in charge of the unit, who may give written permission for nurses to undertake certain tasks. The new Nurses and Midwives Council is working to enhance professional autonomy and recognition, including the right to perform the nursing process independently. In Romania, nursing was a respected profession until 1978, when professional nursing training was abolished. Then its role declined to that of medical assistant, which is the term most commonly used to describe the nurse. There is no sense of autonomy, little teamwork and no understanding of how nursing and medicine use independent but complementary skills. Much of what is normally regarded as a part of the nursing role in other countries is undertaken by doctors, who manage nursing care at the ward level, or is not done at all, especially psychosocial care.

Nevertheless, some fresh thinking is going on about professional roles and functions, and nurses are beginning to develop a new confidence and awareness of their potential. The need to improve the quality of nursing is widely recognized, and it is acknowledged that well educated nurses, midwives and feldshers could help to establish an efficient and effective health care system in all the CCEE and NIS. In the Baltic states, Croatia, the Czech Republic, Hungary, Poland, Slovakia, Slovenia and The Former Yugoslav Republic of Macedonia, nurses are just beginning to be recognized as independent professionals. In the Czech Republic, important legislative changes have resulted in more professional autonomy and an improvement in status. The nurse's role is described as accepting nursing as an activity in which she or he will:

- look for and meet all the biological and social needs of the patient;
- master the methods of the nursing process and use them routinely in all situations;
- consider the patient as a partner and respect his or her rights;
- adopt perfect professional behaviour; and
- make use of information from the social and behavioural sciences to improve communication with patients, families and colleagues.

Of course, all this is far from being universally achieved, but it is a very important sign of the way the wind is blowing.

In theory, if not always in practice, nursing in most of western Europe is in general a professional, independent discipline complementary to those of the other professionals in multidisciplinary teams. Nursing's purpose is usually stated as helping people adopt a healthy lifestyle, enabling them to cope with their health problems, and caring for people of all ages during illness in ways that promote health and healing and minimize disability by responding to the direct needs of the individual, family or community. In all countries, general nurses work in institutions and the community. In most countries a team of nurses has responsibility for total nursing care of the patient or client in hospitals and PHC settings. In a few countries, however, the primary nursing method – in which one nurse is named responsible for the entire care process of one person – is used. (This method is used in both hospitals and the community, and the term primary nursing should not be confused with PHC nursing.)

Some examples show the wide range of philosophies and approaches. In Finland, primary nursing is very widespread. Throughout the Nordic countries, nursing is more or less a comprehensive caring and health promoting activity, with especially well qualified nurses in community care and public health. From being the doctor's assistant with a purely curative function, the nurse in Spain has taken on new tasks for the promotion of health and the prevention of disease and accidents, as well as recuperation and rehabilitation; nursing is moving from the medical model to a way of working based on patient-centred care and problem solving. In Turkey, nurses in theory give preventive, curative and rehabilitative care, but in practice most do not have a proper job description, are subordinate to doctors and have roles in urgent need of clarification. Nurses' formal subordination to medicine remains strong not only in countries such as Greece and Malta, but also in hospitals in countries such as Sweden.

Specialized Roles: Midwifery, Community Nursing and Mental Health Nursing

Increased demands and expectations from patients and the health care system have led to expanded and specialized roles for nurses and midwives in health promotion, disease prevention and care delivery. The broad range of functions within the scope of nursing and midwifery practice today enables the professions to respond flexibly to changing health needs, and creates a rich diversity of roles. In the provision of health care services, good quality and adequate coverage are more important than the professional background of the providers. To deploy services effectively and efficiently by establishing the best mix of grades and skills, however, a clear description is needed of the educational preparation and practice competences of all nursing personnel *(20)*. Although flexibility and diversity are strengths, they may also be a source of conflict between nursing personnel and other health care workers, and sometimes within nursing: the lack of a clear role definition may lead to blurred boundaries and overlap with others' roles. Yet rigid boundaries between and within professions cause conflict and may result in restricted practice. The roles of all health professionals, including doctors, will have to become more flexible, and today's division of labour may change radically in future.

Nowhere is this issue more sharply focused than in the area of nursing specialization. Clinical nurse specialists are experts in a particular aspect of nursing; they demonstrate special clinical expertise, as a result of significant experience, advanced knowledge of a branch or field *(21)*. The outsider, however, may have difficulty in distinguishing an advanced or specialized nursing role from that of a substitute doctor. (The latter role is often characterized as undesirable by professional nursing associations, although the issue should be considered from the viewpoint, not of professional territorialism, but of what will best serve the patient.) Nursing's shift of emphasis to both the community and highly specialized care has led to different views on what services nurses are and are not to deliver.

The examples of the Netherlands and the United Kingdom illustrate some of the differences of opinion. In the United Kingdom, community nurses are increasingly employed by group practices of general medical practitioners (GPs), which are given funds to buy health and social care for their patients. GPs and the NHS recognize the cost–effectiveness of employing nurses to perform certain tasks such as minor surgery, immunization, family planning and some patient consultations. Indeed, doctors are often reimbursed for tasks that nurses actually perform. The role of this "practice" nurse has shown a huge upsurge, although not without critical comment from people who see it as a return to the medical assistant function and deplore the doctor's directly employing the nurse. In the Netherlands, the nursing profession in general opposes this type of role because of the perceived crossing of the boundaries between medicine and nursing and the overlap with an existing occupational group of so-called doctors' assistants. The profession believes that an expanded medical role could damage the caring function of nursing and harm relationships with patients. As a result, the role of specialist nurse practitioner or equivalent was not included in the new law on professions in health care.

Nursing work in Europe is so diverse and broad that the list of specialist roles is almost endless; it changes constantly, reflecting the diversity of needs, health systems, roles, settings and traditions. Some countries have as many as 15 categories of nursing personnel with a wide range of educational preparation. Each country's needs and educational resources determine its range of nursing specialties and the number and preparation of specialists *(20)*. Common examples of specialty areas are maternal and paediatric nursing, mental health and psychiatric nursing, care of the elderly, public health nursing, anaesthesia nursing, emergency and critical care nursing, and rehabilitation.

In addition, some specialists are advanced in various fields of nursing. Examples of advanced practice roles include those of the nurse practitioner, the clinical nursing specialist and the health visitor; they are discussed in Chapter 8. Terms such as specialist and advanced are still controversial and definitions are not universally accepted; most obviously, many midwives define themselves as members, not of a specialist branch of nursing, but of a distinct profession. Advanced practice is generally characterized as:

- specialized in scope
- enhanced in knowledge and skills
- supported by higher education and research
- more independent in practice
- more autonomous in decision-making *(20)*.

Such nurses usually remain in direct patient care and make substantial contributions to the quality of care in primary, secondary and tertiary settings. Moreover, they are able to function as independent and cost-effective practitioners, thus improving coverage to underserved populations. Their deep knowledge and experience mean they have much to offer in health assessment and policy development.

This section discusses three major fields: midwifery, community nursing and mental health or psychiatric nursing. Almost all countries of the European Region have already seen the development of specialized roles in these areas in response to changing needs, such as the growth and the aging of populations, and increases in mental illness. This book cannot cover all specializations; the three examples illustrate some of the key issues relevant to any specialty.

Midwifery

The midwife has a crucial role in reducing maternal and infant deaths and improving the quality of the birth experience. The services of a midwife, however, are not available to all women and progress is still needed in many countries to develop the midwife's role as an independent practitioner skilled in practice, management, critical thinking and leadership.

There is no European consensus on the relationship between nurses and midwives as professions or on the linked issue of midwifery as a separate profession. The positions taken in the debate on these issues have considerable impact on the education and organization of both nurses and midwives. Historical, cultural and sociopolitical circumstances have determined the evolution and status of midwives and their relationship to nurses. In most CCEE and NIS, nearly all deliveries take place in hospital and are usually supervised by doctors. The legal status and functions of midwifery are usually weak and restricted to a role as an obstetric assistant, although there are some notable exceptions. In western and southern European countries, more births take place at home (although the numbers remain small) and midwives have higher status. In general, they are more independent and have a broader role in providing perinatal care. Midwifery usually has a similar status to that of nursing specialties; in countries such as the Netherlands, however, its status and position are higher than those of nursing. The reasons for this include better organization of the profession and midwives' total independence as private practitioners.

In most CCEE, midwives are restricted to providing obstetric and gynaecological care under medical control, and they are not responsible for normal deliveries. As mentioned, nearly all births take place in hospital, and the process is heavily medicalized and often unhealthy and unpleasant for both mother and baby. Countries such as Albania and Bulgaria, however, have a strong midwifery tradition and the midwife is more highly regarded than the nurse; other countries have expanded the role of the midwife. In Albania, midwives are more independent than nurses: they care for women before and after they give birth, visit them at home and conduct all normal deliveries. In Poland, community midwives are responsible for antenatal preventive care on the woman's first clinic visit, home visits during pregnancy (beginning three months later), some deliveries, and care of mother and child until the sixth week after birth. In the former Czechoslovakia, the CNO initiated a review of the role of the midwife. Proposals were drawn up for the reform of legislation to allow midwives more freedom to practise, a new training programme, new delivery techniques and independent practice. In Slovenia, midwifery has recently been recognized as an independent specialty.

In the CCEE, entry requirements for general midwifery training show important variations. In Albania, Croatia, Romania and Slovenia, midwifery training may be undertaken following graduation as a registered nurse. In Albania, a six-month course is replacing the former system of direct entry training. In Bulgaria, the Czech Republic, Poland and Slovakia, midwifery training is completely separate from nursing training, but uses the same entry requirements and education methods (see the section on education, pp. 91–110). In Romania, a three-year midwifery programme was formerly run in conjunction with nursing schools, and all students attended 100 births. In 1978, however, this was replaced by an in-service training programme. Despite Romania's poor standards of maternal and child health, there are no plans to reintroduce midwifery training, owing to the high number of obstetricians. Nevertheless, interest in midwifery is reviving, as shown by the establishment of an NMA.

The situation in the NIS is broadly similar; the midwife provides obstetric and gynaecological care under medical control in hospitals, where most births take place. Home births are more common in rural areas, and at feldsher/midwife posts or stations the midwife has much autonomy and is responsible for antenatal and postnatal care, normal deliveries and health education for mothers and children. All abnormal pregnancies are referred to the district hospital, where doctors assisted by midwives deal with deliveries. The legal status and position of midwives in some NIS have recently improved, partly as a result of the alarming deterioration in maternal and infant health. For example, the health ministry in Uzbekistan described the midwife's role in 1993 as follows. Midwives must be able to take charge of normal births, and provide primary and secondary care to the newborn, emergency care during complications in the course of pregnancy and to the newborn, and initial emergency care in cases of acute disease and accidents. They must carry out simple resuscitation and use modern apparatus for anaesthesia and resuscitation. They must examine pregnant women, including simple investigations of urine and blood, identify risk groups, and treat and care for women giving birth or who are gynaecological patients. Midwives carry out preventive and health education work, prescribe drugs, and monitor infant health and development in the first year.

In all the NIS except Latvia, midwifery education is separate from general nursing education, but has the same entry requirements and is usually taught at the same schools and with the same teaching methods. Training lasts 2½–3½ years, depending on the length of the student's general education.

In most western European countries, midwives are in theory autonomous professionals, conducting normal deliveries and providing antenatal and postnatal care and health education. Their practice includes taking preventive measures and identifying abnormal conditions in mother and child. They may also provide essential treatment to infants, and play an important role in the health education of women, families and the community. Their work encompasses prenatal education, preparation for parenthood, family planning, neonatal care and gynaecological care. In some countries, such as Sweden, midwives may prescribe drugs from a limited list. Midwives may work in public or private hospitals, as freelance practitioners, in local health units or in specialized centres and homes. In the Netherlands, 72% of midwives have their own practice. As a rule, German midwives work independently of the medical profession and are authorized to give instructions to nurses. They also take part in health education in schools and adult education establishments. In the United Kingdom, some midwives have established themselves as independent private practitioners, saying that this gives them a freedom to practise in the mother's and baby's best interests that is too often lacking in institutional settings.

Midwifery's relationship to nursing and its education structures vary throughout western Europe. In Israel, Norway, Portugal, Spain, Sweden and Switzerland, all midwives are registered nurses who then complete a postbasic course. Midwifery training is completely separate from nursing training in Denmark, France, Germany, Greece, Iceland, Italy, Malta and the Netherlands, and takes place in colleges of midwifery. Training normally lasts 3 years, except in Iceland (2 years), France (4 years) and Finland (4½ years). In the United Kingdom, midwifery education is provided through both a direct entry programme and a postbasic course for registered nurses. Direct entry used to be common decades ago, gradually declined and is now reviving. In Belgium, midwifery is a specialty studied after the first year of general nursing training. In Finland, midwifery is one of four nursing specialties, one of which students must choose at the beginning of their studies. In Austria, Ireland, Israel, Norway, Portugal, Spain, Sweden and Switzerland, applicants to midwifery training must be registered general nurses.

Community nursing

The emphasis on community nursing has increased in many countries, starting in the late 1970s and early 1980s. This, together with nurses' change of role from providers of health care to a resource for clients, have brought community nursing into the limelight, even though many countries have a long tradition of nursing service outside hospitals, whether caring for the sick or tackling public health issues. In this book, community nurses is a loose generic term that includes many different roles: feldshers, health visitors, public health nurses, school nurses, occupational health nurses, district nurses and nurse practitioners. As the largest group of primary health care workers, community nurses have an important part to play in the achievement of health for all.

In the CCEE and NIS, relatively few nurses work in the community, owing to the lack of postbasic education, poor status and working conditions, long working hours, low salary and lack of available posts. The nurse is more likely to fulfil the role of medical assistant, carrying out medical procedures or administrative tasks in the health centre or polyclinic. There are a few innovations, as in Hungary, where some district nurses provide home nursing, and mother and child nurses undertake tasks in the community that include family planning and premarital health education. In all countries, role and job content vary widely according to the setting in which the nurse works; in general, nurses in rural areas have far more independence. Owing to the shortage of doctors willing to work in rural areas, medical supervision may be available only part of the time or not at all. When and where doctors are available, nurses usually work as medical assistants, but the scope of their practice can vary enormously within one working day.

In the NIS and some CCEE, the feldsher's role lies somewhere between the traditional roles of the nurse and the doctor. The feldsher is senior to the nurse and has more independence and additional skills. The feldsher carries out health assessments and diagnostic and therapeutic care; performs examinations and tests; recommends treatment plans; provides first aid; and may be allowed to prescribe medication, to diagnose, and to refer patients to doctors if their health does not improve after three days' treatment. Practitioners often combine feldsher and midwifery roles in rural areas, based at village health centres called feldsher/midwife posts or stations. They may also work in emergency services and in factories, where their role focuses on prevention and public health. With the advent of health care reform, however, the role and numbers of feldshers are diminishing in many NIS.

Home nursing is not common in the CCEE and NIS; where community nurses are available, they are more likely to work in health centres or polyclinics, or from their own homes. In rural areas, feldshers and midwives often practise from their homes and have very limited supplies, equipment or opportunities for the safe disposal of clinical waste. Often there is no sterilizing equipment, and disposable items are reused several times. Feldsher/midwife posts and stations are often old, deteriorating, poorly equipped, minimally furnished buildings, sometimes lacking regular electricity or hot running water. Practical difficulties include the lack of transport (the staff may have to walk to their patients, and transport to and from specialist or emergency centres may be restricted), lack of communication (lack of working telephones) and time wasted in searching and queuing for medicines and fuel for heating.

Standards and requirements for the education of nurses working in the community vary widely in the CCEE and NIS. Most countries have no postbasic community training, although short courses may exist. In Poland, for example, a three-month programme is available to nurses with ten years' experience in general nursing. In general, nurses are not seen as needing extra training to work in the community, although there are some examples of postbasic education in health promotion, disease prevention and mother and child care. For example, a three-year course in health visiting is available in Hungary. Some countries offer refresher courses to a limited number of nurses; short specialization courses may be available, but are usually medical in orientation.

In nearly all countries, feldsher training is separate from general nursing education, but has the same entry requirements and takes place in the same schools with the same teaching methods. The age of entry to training is generally around 15–17 years. Training usually lasts 2½ or 3½ years, but many programmes have been discontinued. In general, the training emphasizes preventive care and health education.

Education problems are often compounded by a lack of adequate teaching materials and extremely poor conditions. In many countries, existing books and journals are often outdated and difficult to obtain, and rarely address the needs of nurses and midwives. Many schools of nursing are forced to copy whole textbooks by hand. Some cannot obtain texts in the nurses' own language, and those available are often medical textbooks. Classes may be taught in poorly maintained buildings with no heating or equipment.

In many western European countries, the development or maintenance of community nursing, including home visiting, is described as a priority. While functions such as home visiting are well established in countries such as Denmark, Finland, Iceland, the Netherlands and the United Kingdom, they are relatively underdeveloped in France, Ireland and the Mediterranean countries. The move towards home visiting is being stimulated by demographic changes resulting in a growing elderly population. In most countries, community nursing is a generic term that includes different functions, such as district nursing and health visiting (roles that are combined under the title public health nurse in Ireland), family planning, school nursing, occupational health, psychiatric nursing, mental handicap nursing, paediatric nursing and health education. District nurses and health visitors are usually responsible for the promotion of good health and the prevention of ill health. They work primarily with families needing home care, and those with children under 5 years. Iceland has an extensive home nursing service, and community nurses can care for the elderly population in a flexible way, combining care in the patient's own home with that in a nursing home. School nurses provide health surveillance and health promotion to the school population, and occupational health nurses are concerned with the maintenance of health and a healthy environment in the workplace.

In Finland, one nurse is accountable for care within a specified geographical area; this includes promoting and maintaining the health of the population, preventing illness and providing rehabilitative care, and caring for the dying. In the United Kingdom, nurses have two relatively new roles in PHC: those of the practice nurse and the nurse practitioner. While practice nurses are usually employed by GPs to provide nursing care in the clinic, as mentioned, the nurse practitioner may work in a hospital or the community, is employed by the GP or the health authority, and is authorized to make decisions about patient care and to diagnose, treat and refer patients within the scope of her or his training.

Community nurses most frequently have their base in multidisciplinary health centres or GPs' clinics. Some work from hospital outpatient clinics, minor injuries units, or accident and emergency departments. In some innovative projects, community nurses work in hostels for the homeless, or mobile units such as the psychiatric service offered to the rural population in north-eastern Greece. Community nurses' work is usually managed and supervised by nursing managers, although in the United Kingdom, as mentioned, growing numbers of nurses are employed directly by GPs (but remain accountable to the nursing regulatory body). In practice, community nurses throughout Europe often act on orders from doctors rather than from nurse managers.

The different roles of the community nurse are usually undertaken by qualified nurses with 1–3 years of additional education. In addition, many countries have established refresher courses for community nurses. There are three exceptions. The first is Belgium, where insurance schemes allow private associations to employ social nurses to provide home visiting services; as there is no recognized community nurse training, care is provided by nurses who have had only hospital-based training. The second exception is Austria, where nurses who wish to work in the community may take postbasic training in social–medical nursing; they are considered to be ill prepared for PHC nursing, and other professionals predominate. The third exception is Iceland, where general nursing education prepares nurses to work in both hospital and community settings. This is an ultimate goal of initiatives for nursing education reform in other countries, such as Project 2000 in the United Kingdom.

Mental health nursing[1]

The term mental health nursing is often used not only to describe psychiatric nursing but also to encompass nurses' role in the care of mentally handicapped people. Many countries are not aware of the specific nursing role in either field and, where training exists, it is often very brief.

Mental health nursing is shaped by continuous interaction with its environment. Dramatic changes in social, political and philosophical discourse have not left mental health care and the position of the mental health nurse untouched. Like other nursing roles, it has low status and is still dominated by medicine in some countries. In part, this low status results from that of the patients. Another problem is the difficulty of collecting relevant knowledge about the formal roles and function of nurses in the mental health field. Qualitative and quantitative knowledge about what is actually happening in mental health nursing remains insufficient in many countries.

In the history of mental health, the curative aspect of care dominated services for the mentally ill and mentally handicapped. Doctors and nurses kept their distance from the patient. Illness, disease and mental disabilities were often seen as separate entities, not related to patients as people or to their culture or environment. In this context, knowledge, expertise and power lay in the hands of doctors and their representatives: nurses. Patients were expected simply to accept professional diagnosis and treatment, and nursing interventions were often based not on knowledge about mental health but on delivering care according to doctors' orders. They were often performed without the doctor's supervision or moral and legislative responsibility to patients. Cure-directed care was mostly a solitary process in a tightly organized bureaucracy. Deliberations and consultations within and between multidisciplinary teams almost never occurred.

The environmental conditions in which nurses had to perform their daily duties did not encourage innovation. Nurses worked in badly furnished wards, where hot water or electricity were absent or unreliable and in which many patients were placed. One nurse could be responsible for hundreds of patients, assisted only by unskilled staff who delivered meals and kept the wards clean.

---

[1] This section was written by Bob Keukens, Hans van Pernis and Sascha Olthof.

The same kind of care was given to all patients, without consideration of their individual needs or mental health problems (whether these were neurological illnesses, psychiatric disturbances or mental handicaps). This increased the workload of already overburdened nurses.

In most of the CCEE and NIS, the delivery of mental health care still conforms to this pattern. In the CCEE, the general nurse with minimal postbasic training usually provides mental health nursing; in countries such as Albania, nurses have no role in mental health care. In countries such as the Czech Republic and Hungary, however, the nurse has come to be seen as a professional member of the mental health care delivery team, with her or his own domain, professional responsibilities and specific training.

In all the NIS except the Republic of Moldova, psychiatric care is given by nurses who have undergone general nurse training. Psychiatric and mental health care is concentrated in institutions, and very limited in-service training is available. In the Republic of Moldova, caring for mentally ill people is not part of the role of the nurse; no basic or postbasic training is available. Care for mentally handicapped people is not seen as a nursing task in the NIS. In Kyrgyzstan and elsewhere, nursing standards in mental hospitals are described as low and the staff's role is custodial. Nearly all staff are recruited from the local community.

Curricula for mental health nursing education are still in their infancy in the CCEE and NIS. In the CCEE, specialist training in psychiatric nursing is offered in Hungary, Poland, Slovakia and Slovenia. In Croatia, postgraduate specialization in psychiatric nursing is included in the planned reform of nursing education. In the Czech Republic, the final year of general nurse training has a mental health component; the introduction of a one-year postbasic course is planned. In Albania and Romania, no mental health nurse training is available, although the new curriculum for general nurses in Romania includes both mental health and psychiatric care. A new one-year postbasic curriculum is planned.

In some of the NIS – Belarus, Estonia, Kazakstan, Kyrgyzstan and Latvia – general nursing training gives some coverage of the theory and practice of mental health nursing. Additional in-service training for psychiatric nurses is sometimes available in most countries. For example, in Kazakstan a nurse can in theory take a course lasting 1½–2 months after 5 years' practice.

Secondary prevention and care for mental disorders is part of the nurse's role in all western European countries. Mental health care is often delivered in psychiatric hospitals and/or psychiatric wards, but some countries are moving mental health nursing from institutional care into the community, making the nurse a member of a multidisciplinary team. These countries include Italy, the Netherlands and the United Kingdom.

Where it exists, community mental health nursing ranges from acute care, continuing care and rehabilitation to group therapy and workshops on alcohol and drug use. In many countries, however, health professionals and the public continue to oppose the community approach. Psychiatric nursing is a rather new specialty and most nurses are either general nurses or care assistants.

In many countries, the nurse's role includes the care of people with learning disabilities. This responsibility sometimes lies with social services or education departments; in Austria and Belgium, care for the mentally handicapped is provided mainly by social workers.

At first sight, it seems paradoxical that a dramatic shortage of psychoactive medication is one of the causes for the slow or nonexistent development in mental health. It is paradoxical because the traditional model, oriented towards physical cure, is seen as unwanted. Owing to the introduction of medications such as chlorpromazine, symptoms such as extreme fear, deep depression or psychotic behaviour, about which nothing could previously be done, became more manageable. As a result, psychiatric nursing in western Europe shifted from cure towards care. Indirectly, this development also shifted nurses' attention towards the social environment of the patient, and offered them the chance to create a domain for themselves and gain a certain status. In countries where a shortage of adequate medication makes psychiatric symptoms difficult or impossible to manage, the nursing role is still partly based on the traditional cure model, and includes safeguarding patients and correcting their behaviour.

Shortages of money often preclude a drastic change in the infrastructure of mental health care. Without adequate supplies of medication and better facilities and working conditions, nurses will not have the resources to realize their potential as professionals in mental health care delivery. This has a direct impact on the patients: it helps to prevent their being treated as human beings with different personal characteristics and with illnesses or disabilities related to these characteristics and to the culture and environment. Material changes are required to lead nurses, directly and indirectly, towards a more caring role.

Mental health nurses still have a weak position in the field of health care delivery, mostly owing to the lack of national policies on mental health. As professionals, nurses often disappear under the term "paramedical personnel" in official documents.

In western European countries, specialist training in mental health nursing is offered in Austria, Belgium, Finland, Ireland and the United Kingdom. In Belgium, this starts in the second year of general nurse training. Entry requirements are the same as for general training. In other countries, such as France and Sweden, mental health nursing is part of general training. The three-year programme in Switzerland is giving way to a new programme over a ten-year period that started in 1992. In Denmark, Germany, Greece, Israel, Italy, Luxembourg, Malta, Norway, Portugal and Spain, specialization in mental health takes place after registration as a general nurse, although general training usually deals with some aspects of psychiatric nursing. In the Netherlands, mental health nursing is part of general professional training but is also offered as separate training.

Information on education focusing on nursing care of the mentally handicapped is scarce. In Ireland, the Netherlands and the United Kingdom, basic courses are offered with the same entry requirements as, but separate from, general training. In the United Kingdom, a mental handicap branch course of 1½ years is offered after 1½ years of general nurse training; the course in Ireland lasts 3 years.

Human Resources

WHO promotes the integrated development of health systems and human resources to ensure a supply of personnel with competences relevant to country needs, and balanced according to occupation, specialty and institution. Almost all European countries, however, have imbalances in the supply of nurses, doctors and other health personnel *(22)*. Such imbalances have three dimensions. The numerical dimension involves oversupply or undersupply in relation to a country's needs and resources. The qualitative dimension represents the mismatch between educational preparation and requirements in the workplace. The distributive dimension is geographical, institutional or by specialty. For nursing, the most frequent manifestation of imbalance is undersupply – usually called shortages.

Recognizing the need for better human resource planning, European nurses concluded in 1988 *(1)* that:

> In the light of demographic trends and their implications for the development of primary health care, health manpower policies should be based on health for all and should include:
> – a plan to recruit nursing personnel, drawn up in collaboration with nurses, administrators and politicians and using current manpower data bases;
> – terms and conditions of service that attract and retain qualified nurses, ensure the appropriate use of nursing personnel, and recognize continuing education as a part of career development …

Assessment and planning

The criteria for assessing the balance or imbalance of nursing resources vary between countries and over time, depending on people's perception of health needs, their expectations, the prevalent diseases, the availability of affordable health services, the composition of health care teams, and the cultural and socioeconomic factors that affect people's use of health care services *(22)*. Few countries, however, carry out this type of assessment, which is extremely difficult to make. Tradition and the size of budgets are still the dominant influences.

Human resources planning is an attempt to balance production needs with management needs for personnel. When applied to nursing, its objective is to provide the right number of nurses with the right knowledge, skills and attitudes to carry out the right role in the right place at the right time to achieve the right predetermined goals. Planning cannot be done in isolation, as the work of the nurse is highly interdependent with that of other health professionals and support workers, as well as the level of involvement of the patient, family and informal care givers. Delivering a targeted, cost-effective service requires a careful mixing of disciplines and skills. Planning information is necessary to reorient nursing services from the hospital to the community and to provide re-education at the right time and place. Inaccurate projections of needs for nursing personnel often stem from a lack of the information essential to balance supply with demand. In many countries, such information is unavailable or inaccurate. Even with careful planning, demographic trends, population demands and the state of the labour market can change remarkably quickly, while planning, education systems and recruitment policies cannot.

Human resources policies should be closely linked to overall policy on health services; when this link is weak, problems have greater impact, especially during periods of rapid change. Cost constraints in particular may highlight the shortcomings of traditional methods of human resources planning and deployment, which are based on crude norms such as numbers of staff per hospital bed or simply the previous year's figures. Yet countries focusing on health care reform have been slow to address the need for good human resource planning.

Assessments of present and future needs and the utilization and deployment of nursing personnel are complicated by the variety of staff grouped under this broad heading, and the frequent lack of differentiation between grades, qualifications and competences. In many countries, auxiliary or unqualified staff perform nursing duties and comprise 50–90% of all nursing personnel. They are often included in statistics on nurses, even though they are not competent to perform the duties of a qualified nurse. In addition, aggregated country data usually fail to demonstrate the uneven geographical distribution of health care settings and nursing personnel.

Indications of the number of nurses per bed and per population unit and nurse/doctor ratios are usually the best statistics available, although they fail to compare personnel resources to the need for nursing care. The number of nurses per bed is still used to compare staffing between countries, but the increasing importance of community care and day hospitalization makes such comparisons less significant. The number of nursing personnel (which can also be subdivided by category) per population unit can at least point to the possible human resources available to perform nursing work. Ratios of nurses to doctors cannot match available nursing personnel to the health needs of the population. They give a broad impression of the division of labour in a particular country, but they are also misleading, since people's need for nursing care differs from their need for medical care. The level of joint activity between doctors and nurses is only one of a number of factors requiring consideration. Some analysts argue that no one can rationally defend a situation in which the doctor/nurse ratio is 1 : 3–4 in several northern European countries and 1 : 1.5 in southern and eastern countries. They may be right, but neither can there be any meaningful European norm or universal or lasting indication for each country of the right balance between medical and nursing personnel, since so much depends on the desired outcomes, the job content, the knowledge and skills of each grade of professional staff, traditional and cultural assumptions about health care and professional roles and tasks, health service funds, resource allocation priorities, staff salaries, terms and conditions, and other factors. Finally, the already significant number of part-time workers in some countries and increasing proportions in others (see the section on terms and conditions, pp. 81–91) make it difficult to conduct adequate assessments of present and future needs for education and recruitment.

There is an urgent need to bring statistics on nurses into line with people's need for nursing, rather than institutions' need for nurses. In 1992, as a first step, World Health Assembly resolution WHA45.5 urged Member States to conduct assessments of needs for nursing and midwifery services *(8)*. Since shortages are often accompanied by inappropriate deployment of personnel, the resolution also urged Member States to examine the current roles and utilization of nursing and midwifery personnel. By 1995, a majority of European Member States had complied or said they intended to comply with the resolution. Countries that completed these assessments reported increasing demands for nursing and midwifery services, and shortages of nursing personnel. At the same time, they reported the insufficient or inappropriate use and deployment of staff, with an oversupply in urban areas and a shortage in rural areas. While severe problems continue in the supply and utilization of nursing personnel, countries are clearly recognizing and making greater efforts to deal with them *(22)*.

Numbers and gender issues

The health care systems in the CCEE and NIS, starved of new resources and money to maintain previous standards, are often described as being in crisis. Since the late 1980s, inadequate funding and labour, capital and supply problems have severely disrupted the functioning of health services. The quality of care in state facilities has fallen, and this has not been offset by the increase in costly, sophisticated treatment in private facilities available only to a privileged few. Health service reforms are now under way in most CCEE and NIS, but with little regard for their impact on health personnel other than doctors, whose demands for more money, status and opportunities for private practice are one of the engines of reform. The need to cut costs and acknowledgement of the underuse of hospital beds has led to many closures, with corresponding cuts in staff, especially as many countries still determine staffing levels according to the number of beds. Despite the widely recognized oversupply of doctors and undersupply of well qualified nurses, however, the opportunity was not used to reduce the number of doctors. Usually it was nurses who lost their jobs in local power struggles, thus exacerbating the existing imbalance. So-called middle-level health personnel are poorly deployed and utilized, and a clear division of roles and functions among these nurses, feldshers, midwives and nursing assistants is impossible at present because of inadequate registration systems, poor education, inadequate or nonexistent policies and practices for human resources development, and even the lack of adequate terminology in local languages to describe and differentiate these occupations.

Most CCEE and NIS report severe shortages in qualified nursing staff, regardless of the number of nurses employed. Fig. 1 and 2[2] show large variations between countries. These data suggest that planning of the nursing workforce is usually lacking and, in any case, unrelated to people's need for nursing. As a result, workloads can be very heavy: 1 nurse and 3 support staff having to care for as many as 80 patients is not unusual. Furthermore, real shortages and nurse unemployment go hand in hand in a growing number of countries.

The number of qualified midwives also varies significantly in the CCEE and NIS (Fig. 3 and 4). In general, the number of midwives employed seems to be more closely linked to people's need for midwifery services, as relative numbers follow differences in fertility rates in the CCEE and NIS. These numbers are usually 2–3 times higher in most central Asian republics than they are in, for example, the Baltic states, Croatia and Hungary. Furthermore, countries with large, remote areas, where hospitals are far away and feldsher/midwife posts have a bigger role in perinatal care, seem to employ more midwives than smaller countries with more accessible hospitals.

Fig. 1. Number of nurses per 10 000 population in the CCEE, early 1990s

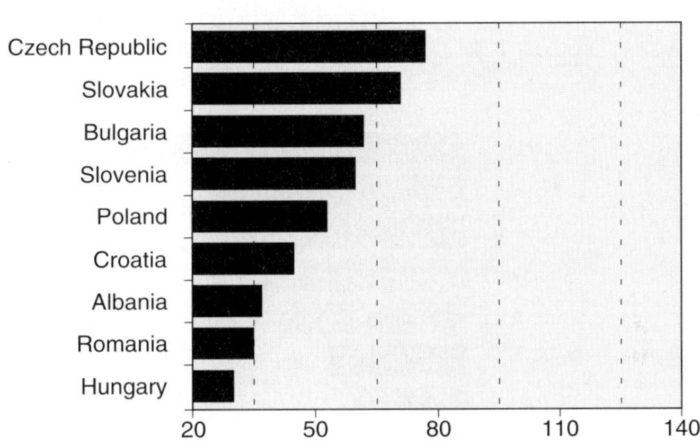

[2] The figures in Chapter 2 give the most up-to-date data available from the WHO Regional Office for Europe and other sources. The figures roughly represent conditions in the early 1990s.

Fig. 2. Number of nurses per 10 000 population in the NIS, early 1990s

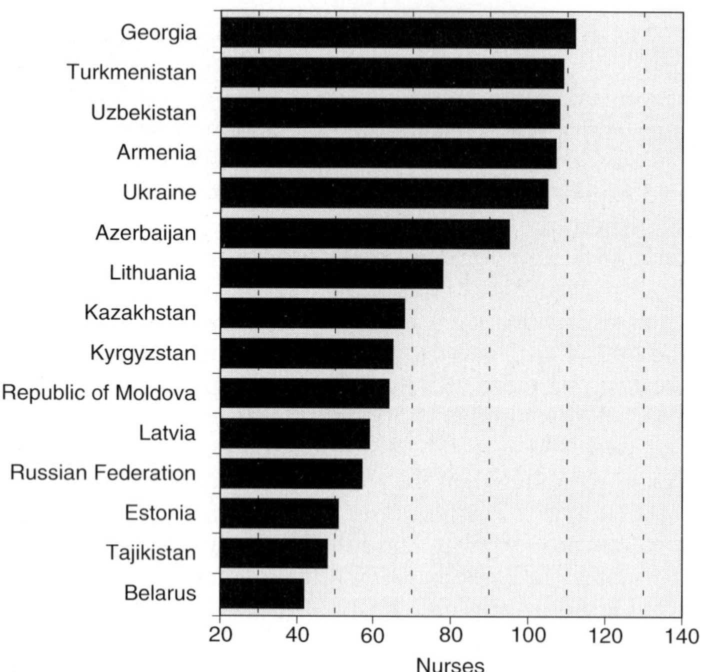

Fig. 3. Number of midwives per 10 000 population in the CCEE, early 1990s

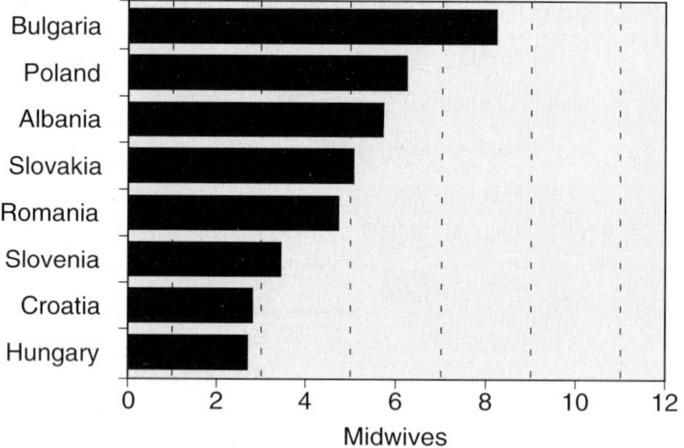

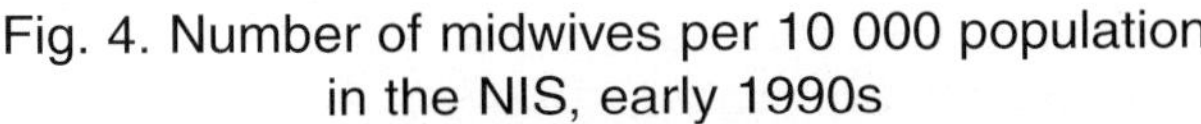

Fig. 4. Number of midwives per 10 000 population in the NIS, early 1990s

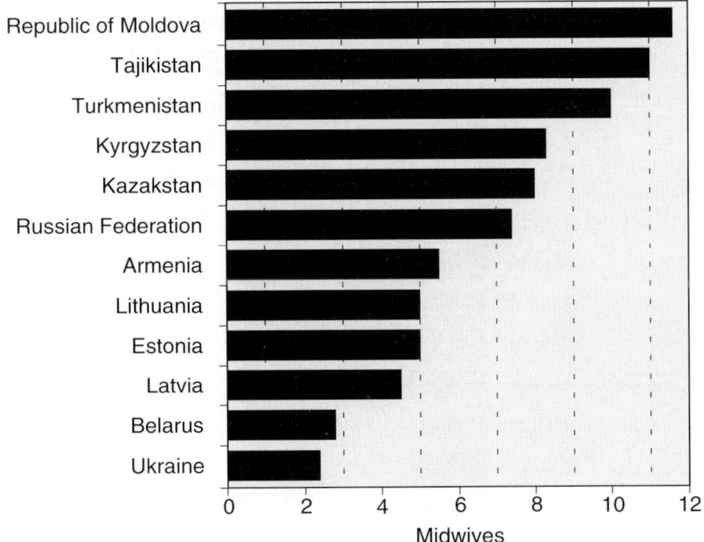

In all the CCEE and NIS, nursing is women's work and shares the characteristics of other female-dominated occupations: low pay, low status, poor working conditions, few prospects for promotion and poor education. Gender ratios underline these statements: women comprise 90–99% of the total nursing population in the CCEE and NIS (see Fig. 5). Within the nursing profession, however, the feldshers – the most independent, best qualified and most senior nurses – are mostly men. These figures indicate not only that the nursing profession as a whole suffers from gender discrimination, but also that women do not have the same status and career prospects as their male colleagues.

In western Europe's established market economies, health care delivery and financing and, increasingly, health professional training are mixtures of public and private initiatives, making human resource planning even more complex. The proportion of registered nurses working in the private sector varies, being 15% in France and 4% in Finland. Although public organizations and institutes are the main employers of nursing and other health care personnel in all countries, private practice is gaining ground. This trend was reinforced by both economic recessions in the 1980s and early 1990s, and ideological shifts in the role of government in health care. Almost without exception, responsibility for health care purchasing and delivery in the public sector has been de-

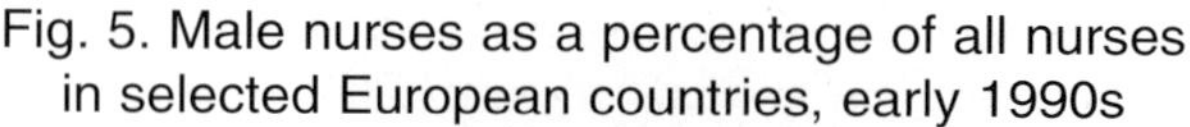
Fig. 5. Male nurses as a percentage of all nurses in selected European countries, early 1990s

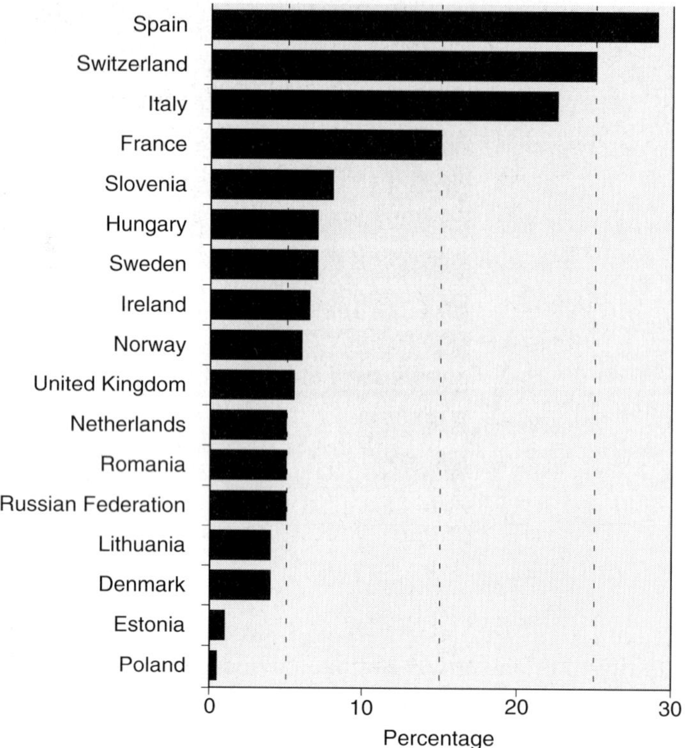

centralized to regional or municipal health authorities, who are almost all under strong financial pressure. As a result, more emphasis is given to sharing this responsibility between the public and private sectors, with a growing role for insurance companies and patients or clients in the financing of health care, and more private initiatives in the delivery of care, especially in hospitals and nursing homes.

The numbers of qualified nurses in western Europe vary enormously, ranging from 8 per 10 000 population in Turkey to 137 in Norway (Fig. 6). In general, the ratios follow a north–south divide, with more nurses per 10 000 population in northern countries (usually 70–90) than in the south (usually 20–40). The number of nurses appears more close-

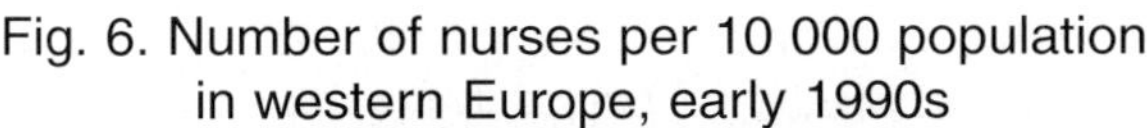

Fig. 6. Number of nurses per 10 000 population in western Europe, early 1990s

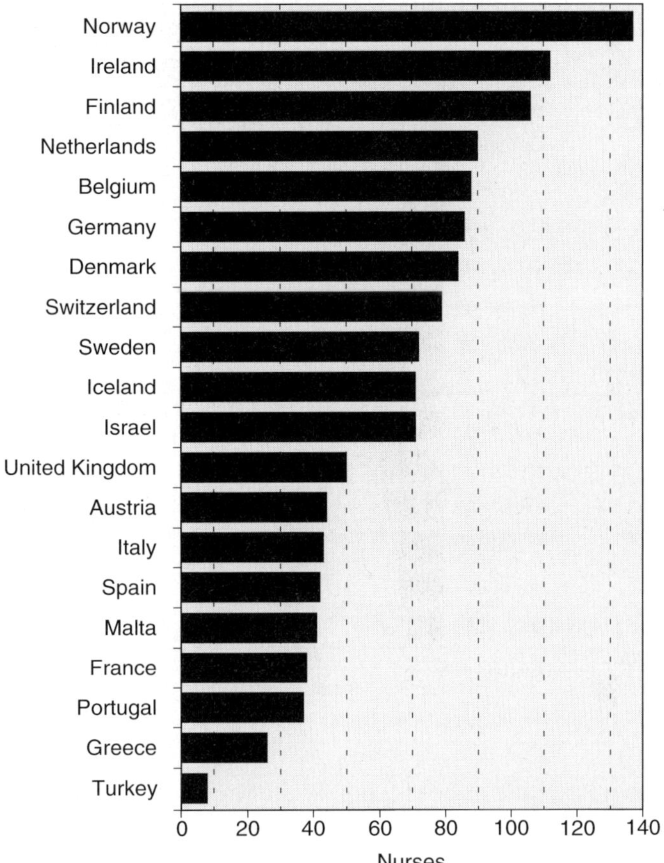

ly correlated with income-related indicators, such as gross domestic product (GDP) per head, than with health care needs. For example, shortages of nurses, especially in rural areas, are reported in Greece, Italy, Malta, Portugal and Turkey. Difficulties in recruiting qualified staff are common throughout these countries, mainly owing to poor pay, poor working conditions and lack of career opportunities.

The number of qualified midwives per unit of population throughout western Europe (Fig. 7) seems to have no relation to fertility rates, a country's health care system or the number of nurses employed, although these factors vary widely. A country such as the Netherlands, where midwives have heavy responsibility for perinatal care and many

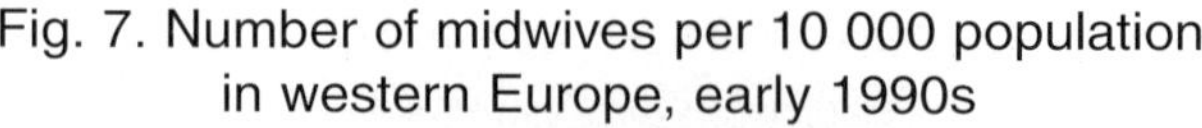
Fig. 7. Number of midwives per 10 000 population in western Europe, early 1990s

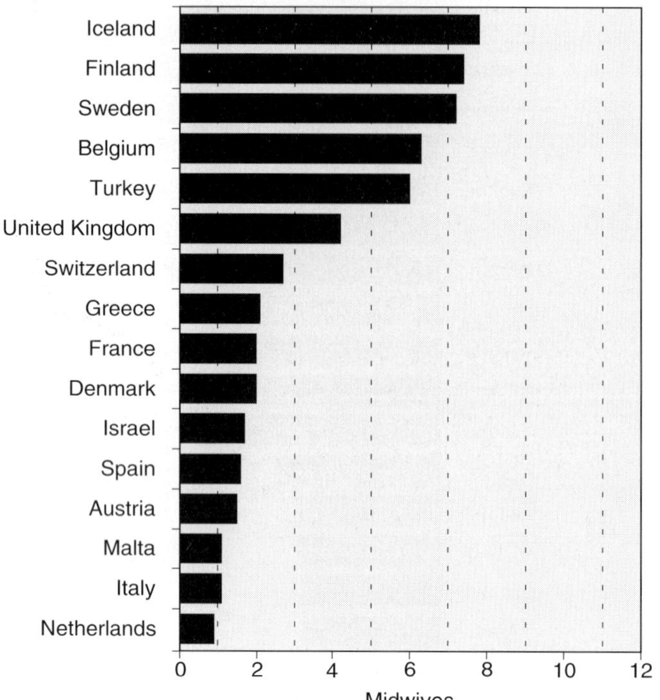

deliveries take place at home, has less than 1 midwife per 10 000 population, while in Belgium, Sweden and the United Kingdom the number is 4–8 times higher. These huge differences can in no way be fully explained by variations in countries' demographic characteristics and geography, or in midwives' responsibilities, roles and functions.

With regard to gender issues, female predominance in nursing is evident in all western European countries, where usually less than 10% of the workforce is male (Fig. 5). Exceptions are Italy, Malta, Spain and Switzerland, where men comprise about a quarter or more of the total. In Spain, the reasons could include the bar on recruitment to medical education introduced in the 1970s. This forced many men who intended to study medicine to choose another profession, or to take a nursing course first and then to apply again for medicine. Another explanation could be general shifts in the labour market in the 1970s, including mass unemployment in many traditionally male occupations. In some countries, too, nursing today presents relatively more career opportunities, including management and research, that enhance its appeal to men and subvert its traditional feminine image. Status, working conditions and salaries are poor in many countries, especially for female nurses, since a disproportionately high number of men occupy nursing positions with better pay and higher status. In some countries, men are still paid more than their female colleagues in the same jobs.

Recruitment and retention

The number of nurses worldwide is falling, and recruitment and retention are major concerns in many countries. Unless this is taken into consideration as part of a country's overall health policy, the number of nurses may continue to fall, with serious consequences for health care coverage and quality. The factors that affect recruitment and retention are complex and interrelated, and the accurate assessment of cause and effect requires a range of demographic, educational and environmental information. Two main issues, however, dominate all discussions about choosing nursing as a career and staying in it: working conditions and the image of nursing *(20)*.

Good working conditions positively affect the recruitment and retention of nursing personnel, especially in underserved areas, as well as the quality of practice. Working conditions are defined here as including not only the facilities in a workplace, but also health and safety issues, hours of work, workload, the conditions in which nursing personnel and their families have to live their daily lives, and less tangible but perhaps equally important factors such as the quality of workplace relationships with colleagues and managers, and the way in which the organization handles work-related stress.

These conditions appear to be especially poor in rural areas, where, paradoxically, health care providers are most needed *(23)*. The professional isolation often experienced in rural postings is also significant. The presence of other health personnel with a team-based approach greatly enhances both the quality of care and the motivation of team members. Job satisfaction is greater where the local community is both encouraged and empowered to increase social support for nursing personnel, and contributes actively to the planning, delivery and evaluation of local health care services. This can give the community nurse a status akin to the traditional one of village healer, elder or wise woman, which also gives satisfaction. Nurses who come from the community in which they work, understand its ways and speak its language are more likely to be satisfied and to work well than those who are posted to places where they are strangers and perhaps marginalized or mistrusted.

Pay remains a key factor for nursing globally. Nurses are poorly paid in most countries (see the next section). Low pay is accompanied by few incentives or benefits and a lack of career structure. In addition, nursing personnel are often sought after in other areas of work; if these have better pay and conditions, it is little wonder that they leave the profession. Some countries overcome local recruitment problems or circumvent collective wage agreements by purchasing services on a contractual basis, for example, from profit-making nursing agencies. Another problem is the lack of financial incentives to remain in clinical posts. Some countries where nurses are in long-term government service are starting to explore whether their continued employment should be contingent on the quality of their performance *(19)*, and to introduce professional structures that reward clinical expertise as highly as education or management skills.

Pay, conditions of work and the level of autonomy are important factors that affect the image of nursing. Others no less important are the cultural and social values relating to so-called women's work and work that necessitates close contact with blood, excreta and human bodies. The image of nursing is poor in many countries, and is typically linked to the level of true respect and value for women in general. Such a negative image has long-term effects on the quality of nursing, not least because able students who have a choice of career may be unlikely to choose nursing. A radical change of image is not likely to occur without the development of a new social consciousness that values care and care giving.

A 1995 WHO Expert Committee *(20)*, addressing problems of recruitment and retention, recognized two significant trends: the growing privatization of many health care services and the migration of nurses. As mentioned, health care systems in many European countries, and indeed throughout the world, are currently engaged in reform initiatives. Many countries have adopted a strategy of greater private-sector involvement in the delivery of health care. The private sector has traditionally been involved mainly in the delivery of secondary and tertiary care, which reinforces the need for governments to continue to reallocate resources to PHC. As the private sector grows, governments should develop regulatory, quality assurance and monitoring mechanisms that establish standards of care, guarantee acceptable working conditions, and ensure equity and access to health services for vulnerable groups such as the elderly, the urban and rural poor and the mentally ill.

Migration is the other important trend. Nursing policy has been influenced by the aim of facilitating freedom of movement of professionally qualified people within the EU through mutual recognition and harmonization of qualifications. Although the volume of migration is still low, nurses in the European Region increasingly move from poorer to richer countries seeking better employment opportunities. The EC directives on the mutual recognition of nursing and midwifery qualifications appear to have had relatively little impact on labour mobility, although this may change.

The movement of nurses within the CCEE and from the CCEE to western European countries, mainly Austria and Germany, is a new phenomenon facilitated by political change, armed hostilities in some areas and the shortages of qualified nurses in many countries. Many hospitals in the west actively recruit the best-qualified nurses from neighbouring CCEE. Most of them do not possess the credentials to be registered for practice in the host countries, so they may work as nursing assistants, thus providing a cheap service. This in turn may undermine nursing's position in negotiating collaborative agreements on terms and conditions of work. While free movement is a basic human right, migration poses serious challenges to both labour-exporting and labour-importing countries. Poor countries may gain from the money sent home, but many CCEE are experiencing a deterioration in health, leading to an increase in people's need for nursing. The migration of well educated nurses to neighbouring countries represents a nursing brain drain that societies can ill afford. Moreover, countries that import foreign nurses should prepare them to provide care that is culturally and linguistically appropriate, yet few do anything to tackle this challenge.

Problems with matching supply and demand for nursing staff are reported throughout the European Region. Shortages of well educated nursing staff and difficulties in recruiting suitably qualified nurses are common in the CCEE and NIS. The main reasons for difficulties in recruiting newly qualified nurses are low status, poor salaries and bad working conditions. Furthermore, nurses are migrating from rural to urban areas and from the public to the private sector. All this affects initial recruitment into the profession. For example, Hungary reports a low number of applicants for training; many entrants lack the basic requirements. In many situations, especially in the NIS, auxiliaries are the only staff available to fill qualified posts. High turnover rates, sometimes up to 50% of the whole workforce annually, are reported in Azerbaijan, Belarus, Georgia, the Republic of Moldova, the Russian Federation, Tajikistan and elsewhere. Some countries, however, report no problems in the recruitment of new nurses. For example, the World Bank *(23)* states that in Albania the health system is well staffed, there is an oversupply of applicants and, despite high emigration rates, nurse graduates may have difficulty finding jobs.

Recruitment and turnover ratios vary significantly in western Europe and are highly correlated with status and working conditions, as well as with demographic factors, government policy and conditions in the national and local labour markets. The picture can also change relatively fast, making generalization or the mapping of trends difficult. Some countries report shortages of nurses and nursing students and high turnover rates. Elsewhere, cuts in health service spending, reducing the number of posts, have mopped up surplus staff, although recruitment for specialist posts may still be a problem. A recent study *(24)* suggested that shortages in the supply of nursing personnel in the EU do not seem to be as widespread as frequently assumed.

In Ireland and the United Kingdom, where the status of nurses is relatively high, the number of applicants for training was, until recently, greater than the number required. In Israel, however, which also has a reportedly high status of nurses, the number of applicants for training every year is satisfactory, and nurse unemployment is nearly absent. In addition, turnover rates in these countries are relatively low: 3% in Ireland and 7% in England, for example. Nevertheless, England is experiencing a shrinking nursing workforce, owing to cuts in posts and problems with the professional image of nursing, as well educated young people confront a wide range of career choices. Some countries, such as Iceland, Norway, Spain and Switzerland, report no significant problems in the recruitment of nurses. In Germany and Spain, imbalances in the recent past have been corrected. Other countries, such as France, Greece, the Netherlands, Portugal and Turkey, report shortages of nurses and students, mainly due to relatively poor status, pay and working conditions. Their turnover rates are also usually much higher: 17% of nurses in the Oslo region in Norway and 20% in mental health care in the Netherlands, for example.

In Italy, the number of students increased considerably as a result of campaigns to enhance the public image of nursing by providing more economic assistance and job security. On the other hand, very little has been done to retain nurses in hospitals, and a nurse spends an average of about ten years in the hospital service. Reasons include the lack of career possibilities, burn-out caused by overwork, and low salaries. The number of training places was recently reduced, yet there are shortages of nurses, often linked to poor organization of the work and inappropriate use of nursing resources.

Some governments, such as those of Austria, Germany and Malta, are taking steps to improve the status and attractiveness of nursing. In Austria, this includes state subsidies to hospitals to improve the ratio of qualified to unqualified personnel. In Germany, the salaries of all nurses were increased by 3.5% in 1993. At the same time, the salaries of nurses in the former German Democratic Republic have been raised to 80% of those of nurses in other regions. The shortage of nursing professionals, which existed both in regional terms and in different areas of the profession, has been markedly reduced since 1990; the attractiveness of the profession to young people has improved substantially in recent years, and outflow has decreased, owing to the rises in salary, improvements in other working conditions and the recent recession in the country. Malta faces a problem in recruiting and retaining qualified staff and is trying to attract foreign nurses. Plans are emerging that include better salaries and better facilities to attract young recruits and to retain those already in the profession, especially married women.

In Turkey, the number of qualified staff is considered too low, in part because of poor working conditions, which vary between institutions and in some cases prevent nurses from delivering an acceptable level of care. Some regions report particular problems with absenteeism. Greece and Portugal also face a significant shortage of health personnel, particularly nurses.

Terms and Conditions of Work

Nurses' terms and conditions of work – such as status, pay, working hours and working conditions, shift work, and employers' personnel policies – exert an important influence on the quality of nursing and health care in the Region. As shown in the previous section, unfavourable terms and conditions are frequently given as reasons for problems with recruitment and retention. Many factors contribute to nurses' disadvantageous position. First, nursing in general shares the characteristics of other traditionally female occupations: low pay, low status, poor working conditions, few prospects for promotion and poor education. Second, the real value of the profession is not recognized in many countries, and lags behind people's sharply increased needs and expectations. Third, the heterogeneous character of the profession hinders its taking a strong and powerful position in relation to government, employers and the medical profession. Furthermore, the current economic situation, and the avowed determination of most countries to reduce or check the rise in health care spending, make it difficult to secure greater attractions, including better pay and conditions *(19)*.

International standards

Nursing personnel are covered by ILO conventions and recommendations, which lay down general standards for all employees, relating in particular to working conditions and equality of opportunity. In view of the particular conditions of nursing, however, the need for specific standards to complement these instruments soon became apparent. In 1944, the recommendation on medical care stated that the working conditions of doctors and members of allied professions should be designed to relieve them from financial anxiety by providing adequate income during work, leave, illness and retirement *(4)*. More recently, in response to a report on the employment and working conditions of nursing personnel, ILO Recommendation 157 was adopted in 1977 *(4)*. It proposes measures to offer nursing personnel reasonable career prospects through a grading and remuneration structure. This should be based on:

- a classification of the levels of qualification and judgement required, the authority to make decisions, the complexity of the relationship with other functions, and the level of responsibility; and
- on a classification of nursing personnel within a limited number of categories determined by reference to education and training, level of functions and authorization to practise.

Income

ILO Recommendation 157 contains an entire chapter devoted to remuneration *(4)*. Nearly 20 years after its adoption, these provisions are still the benchmarks to assess individual countries' performance. It contains the following provisions.

1. Nurses' pay should be fixed at levels commensurate with their socio-economic needs, qualifications, responsibilities, duties and experience, taking account of the constraints and hazards inherent in the profession.
2. Levels of remuneration should be such as to attract people to the profession and retain them, and should also bear comparison with those of other professions requiring similar or equivalent qualifications and carrying similar or equivalent responsibilities.
3. Levels of remuneration for nursing personnel having similar or equivalent duties and working in similar conditions should be comparable, whatever the establishments, areas, or sectors in which they work.
4. Remuneration should be adjusted from time to time to take into account variations in the cost of living and rises in the national standard of living.
5. Nursing personnel who work in particularly arduous or unpleasant conditions should receive financial compensation.

6. Finally, work clothing, medical kits, transport facilities and other supplies required by the employer or necessary for the performance of the work should be provided by the employer and maintained free of charge.

None of the CCEE or NIS complies with the ILO Recommendation. In all CCEE, nurses' wages are reported to be inadequate or poor in absolute terms. For example, the wages of nurses in Hungary (equivalent to US $1500–1600 a year in 1994) and Romania (equivalent to US $300–400 a year in 1994) are just above the poverty line. Nurses' wages usually compare very poorly with national averages. For example, a Slovene nurse earns the equivalent of US $5500 a year, while GDP per head was US $8000 in 1995. Rapid inflation in many countries has further eroded the real value of salaries, and many nurses cannot make ends meet on salaries alone. This forces them to do overtime, take an additional job or search for informal ways of earning money. Some countries, however, report improvements. For example, nurses in the Czech Republic won higher salaries, moving from the 3–5 tariff range to the 6–8 tariff range in the new wage system (which has 12 tariff points) initiated by the 1992 law on wages. Different rates of pay take account of nurses' postgraduate achievements.

The picture in the NIS is similar and often worse. In all countries, nurses' income is low or very low (Table 5). Pay in the health sector is usually 50–75% of the national average, and nurses earn relatively little compared to other health care professionals. In some countries, staff may be paid nothing at all for months on end. Nurses' low income is affecting morale and productivity; in the Russian Federation it generated unprecedented strike action. Government moves to allow local hospitals to establish their own pay scales, sparking fears of a downward wage spiral, provoked mass protests in Estonia in 1995.

Table 5. Nurses' income in selected CCEE and NIS, 1991–1994

Country	Monthly income (US $)
Tajikistan	3
Republic of Moldova	10–22
Russian Federation	15
Lithuania	15–20
Estonia	42–51

In most western European countries, nursing personnel employed by the public sector are paid according to regulations or collective labour agreements between employers and trade unions. With a few exceptions, such as Spain, nurses working in the private sector are better paid than their public-sector colleagues, although that is more likely to be the case in an acute hospital than in a nursing home for the elderly, and data not only vary widely but are difficult to collect. Nurses' wages are usually somewhat lower than those of other professions requiring similar education levels. In Denmark, for example, a nurse's salary is comparable to that of a skilled craftsman. Nurse managers and teachers have higher salaries, as do those in specialist fields such as infection control, psychiatry and health visiting. Nursing auxiliaries and assistants are often among the lowest paid workers in society.

Wages in most countries are about the national average or somewhat below, except in Austria, Belgium, Greece, Italy and Turkey, where they are much lower. In Spain, for example, the general nurse's average 1992 salary of nearly 2.4 million pesetas (equivalent to US $15 000) is similar to those of other workers of the same level. Salary levels differ between nurses in specialized care and those in PHC, in favour of the latter. In the United Kingdom, a ward sister with a starting salary of US $20 500 (1992) earned 87% of the average national wage, while in Ireland the starting salary of a qualified nurse compares quite favourably with those of other health professionals; on the other hand, nurses are not paid according to their responsibilities and differentials are very poor. In Italy, nurses receive a basic salary that is regarded as inadequate, even though numerous supplements are paid (for particular duty hours, overtime, rotation, hazardous work, etc.). There is little difference between the salaries of auxiliaries and registered nurses, and little career development. The annual salary is the equivalent of US $12 800, about the same as an average office worker. In the Netherlands, the starting salary of a general nurse is equivalent to some US $18 000 a year (2584 guilders per month in 1994) and is significantly lower than that of comparable professions. A specialist nurse may expect at least US $6000 more a year.

Nurses' salaries in some countries, such as Belgium, France, Germany, Greece, Italy and the United Kingdom have, however, risen or been adjusted during the 1990s to improve recruitment. In a few countries remuneration increased considerably; for example, some specialist nurses in Germany received an increase of 30%.

In general, women's average salaries are lower than those of men in similar jobs, although the picture varies between countries and according to salary and career structures, differentials between grades and qualifications, and other factors. For example, the average differential between men's and women's pay in Sweden is 1.6% in favour of men. The average pay of female nursing assistants and auxiliaries employed by county councils, however, is slightly higher than that of men. In contrast, male nurses in the United Kingdom earn 21% more than female nurses, and nursing auxiliaries show an even greater differential: women earn only 55% of men's salaries. Although there is equal pay legislation, disproportionately more male nurses hold better paid jobs, and many more women work part time to combine a job and child care.

A study conducted by ILO in 1994 *(19)* reported that pay is perceived as unsatisfactory worldwide. This is felt all the more keenly as the constraints and demands of the work are heavy and made even heavier by staff shortages. Nurses' demands for better pay relate first to basic salary, which is manifestly inadequate in relation to those of comparable professionals such as teachers, and to continuing efforts to upgrade nursing's social and professional status. The demands also address special allowances, particularly for working overtime and stressful or unusual hours, which considerably increases the arduousness of the work, and for shift work, with its special constraints. Nurses also insistently demand a guaranteed level of purchasing power or its maintenance, particularly in countries where inflation is high. In a number of countries, nurses and trade unions are highlighting problems arising from excessive pay differentials within the profession, which not only cause discontent but also aggravate staff shortages in the worst paid sectors.

Nurses' growing demands have been marked in recent years and have featured in well publicized pay campaigns in many countries. Sometimes these have included strikes or other forms of withdrawal of labour, at odds with the traditional image of nurses and therefore all the more noticeable. In 1995 alone, lengthy pay disputes in Denmark, Sweden, the United Kingdom and elsewhere caught the mass media's attention.

Working hours and leave entitlement

ILO Recommendation 157 *(4)* proposes that:

- in countries where the normal working week exceeds 40 hours, it should progressively be reduced to 40 hours for nursing personnel, without loss of salary;
- overtime and work performed on public holidays should be compensated, and compensation may take the form of an addition to salary;

- work performed at inconvenient or stressful hours other than on public holidays, and also shift work, should be compensated by an addition to salary; and
- exposure to special risks should give rise to financial compensation.

All CCEE and western European countries have complied with the ILO recommendations on nurses' working hours, at least in theory. The average working week varies widely in the Region (Fig. 8), although it is 37–39 hours in most countries. The shortest full-time working week is found in Portugal. Nurses in all NIS officially work 41 hours over 6 days, although some working in poor conditions may have a limited day of 5.5 hours. The public health law limits the working day to 12 hours.

In general, nurses employed by the private sector have a longer working week than those in public institutions. For example, the average working week of private sector nurses is 39.4 hours in Spain and 40 hours in Greece, exceeding that of public sector nurses by some 2.5 hours.

In some countries, a significant proportion of the nursing population works part time: Belgium (25–52%), the Netherlands (58%), Sweden (41%) and the United Kingdom (34%). In most countries, however, opportunities for working part time are restricted, especially in the CCEE and NIS and some southern European countries. In Greece, for example, only nurses in the private sector may work part time. Consequently the number of part-time jobs in these countries forms only a very small proportion of total nursing posts.

On the other hand, working overtime is a common, almost institutionalized, feature of nursing in many countries. Overtime is a subject of special importance, particularly for hospital staff, because of the need to ensure a continuous service in the interest of the patients and because of staff shortages. Overtime is very often used to compensate for structural shortages of staff, rather than to cope with occasional peak workloads or staff sickness. Compensation regulations for overtime differ widely but are based on granting time off or overtime pay, or combining the two. Where staff shortages are acute, employers often prefer to provide compensation in cash, and this involves payment at a higher hourly rate in many countries. This is in accordance with ILO Recommendation 157, and with the 1962 ILO Recommendation 116 on the reduction of hours of work for all professions *(4)*, which urges that:

- all hours worked in excess of normal hours be deemed to be overtime, unless they are taken into account in fixing remuneration in accordance with custom;

- limits be fixed to the total number of hours of overtime that can be worked during a specified period;
- overtime be remunerated at a rate not less than 25% higher than that applicable to normal hours of work.

In practice, differences between countries in overtime payment rates give rise to considerable variation in the real rate of payment for overtime worked. Switzerland, for instance, remunerates overtime, when not compensated by time off or a rest period, exactly 25% higher than the rate for normal hours of work, when worked on a weekday between 7 a.m. and 8 p.m., and at 150% in other cases. In Spain, all overtime is

Fig. 8. Average number of nurse's working hours per week in selected European countries, early 1990s

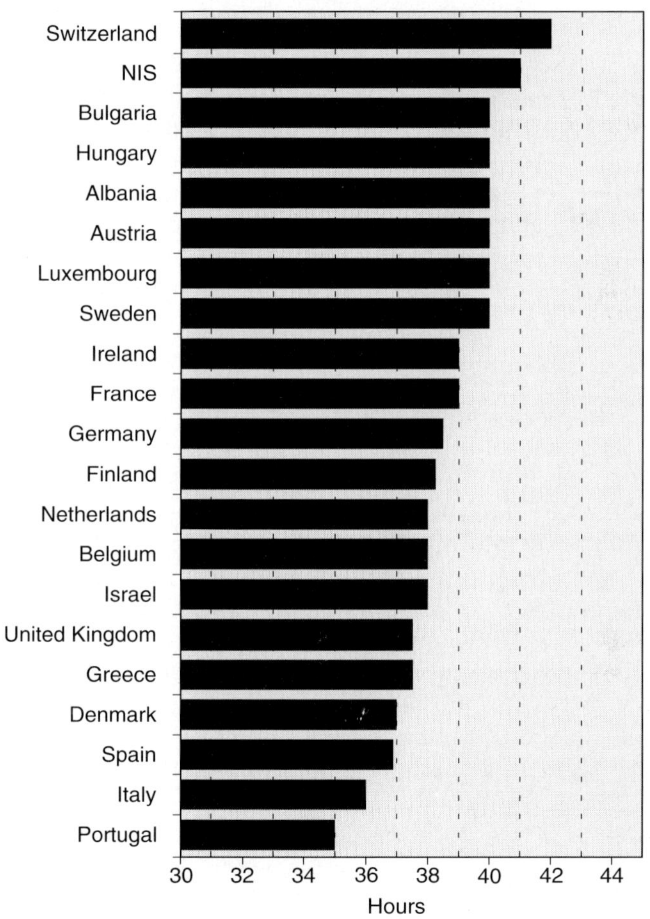

compensated at 175%. In the Netherlands, time off is the normal compensation but, when additional payments are made, the rate is 138% for overtime on weekdays after 6 p.m. In Sweden, the first two hours of overtime in any month are paid at 180% of the normal rate and all additional hours at 140%.

With regard to the second provision, few countries restrict overtime. In the public sector in France, the maximum permissible number of hours of overtime is 20 per month. Italy applies a yearly maximum of 50 hours. In Sweden the restriction is twofold: 50 hours per month and 200 per year.

Countries show similar large differences in compensation for working night shifts, weekends and public holidays *(19)*. Paid annual leave entitlement and public holidays also vary widely (Table 6), although most countries report between 24 and 27 annual leave days and some 10 public holidays.

Table 6. Annual paid leave entitlements and public holidays in selected European countries

Country	Paid leave (days)	Public holidays
Austria	25	
Belgium	22	
Bulgaria	16	5
Denmark	25	10
Germany	26–30	
France	30	11–13
Finland	24	
Greece	22	
Ireland	32	8
Israel	26	
Italy	30	6
Luxembourg	25	
Malta	25	
Netherlands	24	7
NIS	24	
Portugal	22	10
Spain	30	14
Sweden	24	
Switzerland	20	
United Kingdom	25	10–12

Furthermore, the length of fully paid maternity leave varies considerably, as shown by the following examples:

- in Switzerland, nurses are entitled to a minimum of 8 weeks' maternity leave;
- in Israel, maternity leave is 12 weeks; a nurse may be relieved from working night shifts after 20 weeks of pregnancy; and on return to work after giving birth, a nurse's regular shift is shortened by 1 hour for 1 year;
- in Malta, maternity leave is 13 weeks, which can be extended by a year's unpaid child-care leave;
- in France, maternity leave is 16 weeks, with 28 weeks granted as from the third child;
- in Denmark, maternity leave is 8 weeks before and 14 weeks after birth;
- in Italy, maternity leave is granted at full salary for 2 months before and 3 months after the birth, after which the mother may take a further 6 months' leave at reduced salary during the child's first year, as well as unpaid leave until the child reaches the age of 3 years;
- in the Netherlands, nurses are entitled to 6 months' fully paid maternity leave, to be taken as they choose;
- in Bulgaria and Poland, nurses and midwives are entitled to 3 years' partly paid maternity leave;
- in the NIS, posts are sometimes kept open – and therefore unfilled – for years awaiting the mother's return; this causes major problems, especially in countries where fertility rates are high, such as the central Asian republics.

Paternity leave is a growing phenomenon but is usually unpaid when granted at all. Only in the Nordic countries can one really speak of parents' leave. In Denmark, male nurses have the right to 2 weeks' paid leave in the first 14 weeks after birth. The right to a further 10 weeks' leave is granted to either the mother or the father, but not both. In Sweden, parents are entitled to 15 months' paid leave on the birth of a child, which can be shared between the father and mother and can be taken any time before the child reaches the age of 8.

Working conditions

As mentioned above and reported by the ILO in 1994, nurses everywhere complain frequently about the difficulties experienced in their normal professional work *(19)*, and these difficulties form the basis of some of the demands of professional associations and trade unions. For instance, a reduction in normal working hours is being urged with increasing insistence. The deterioration of working conditions, resulting from chronic shortages of staff and from shortages of materials and equipment, is also often highlighted. Continuing staff shortages unquestionably add to the normal workload, aggravated when those absent for varying periods (on holiday, or sick or maternity leave) are not replaced. The remaining personnel are thus forced not only to work harder, but to resort to practices that may involve risk for both patient and nurse. In some countries, the shortage of auxiliary staff or an oversupply of doctors forces nurses to perform lower-level tasks that are not normally their responsibility; in others, shortages mean that nursing duties are assigned to less qualified personnel. In addition, when nurses also have administrative duties and an institution places a higher value on completing paperwork than on caring for patients, they may have to delegate their primary responsibilities for practice to support workers, thus jeopardizing the quality of care. Excessive workload also leads to neglect of supervisory responsibilities for junior staff and students, and to situations in which daily practice falls far short of what is taught in training colleges.

Finally, nurses deplore the lack of attention paid to the predominance of women in the profession. Overwork and stress are difficult for any employee to tolerate and should not be accepted, but these problems are particularly acute for nurses who are also caring for children and/or elderly relatives: the responsibilities of the so-called double shift – home and work – which few men share. Rather than acknowledging that nurses are a mainly female workforce, and taking account of this in policies and practice, many employers appear oblivious to the special situation of and demands placed on working women. The lack of workplace childcare facilities, the lack of flexible working hours and practices to take account of family obligations, the insufficient attention to developing opportunities for satisfying part-time work, and the inadequacy of protection during pregnancy are just a few examples of this gender blindness. These issues are often mentioned as reasons why nurses leave the profession, and they should be tackled not only to improve women's and families' rights, but also to avoid the further drift of nursing personnel towards occupations and employers that offer better working conditions.

Trade unions have a special role in encouraging employers to enforce the ILO recommendations at the national level. In all European countries, nursing personnel are represented by general trade unions, trade unions of health care personnel and/or professional organizations with labour relations functions. As mentioned, nurses often have a choice between organizations of each type, and choose to join more than one organization in some countries. Representation usually exists at the different levels where working conditions are examined and determined (federal or national, regional, cantonal, local levels or individual institutions). Many different trade unions and professional organizations take part in collective bargaining in many countries. For example, nursing personnel are represented by four trade union confederations in Italy and six unions in Spain. In the United Kingdom, nurses are represented by nine organizations, including the Royal College of Nursing, which acts as both a professional organization and a trade union, and UNISON, a giant public-sector union. Very few organizations can truly claim exclusive representation of nursing personnel. In some countries, the difficulties of multiple representation are partly overcome by establishing a consortium or "staff side" of organizations that reaches consensus in order to present a united front to management and thus to bargain more effectively.

The ILO recommendations have been signed by all the European Member States of WHO and should provide both the framework for and the basis of collective bargaining between governments, employers and employees, regardless of the formal inequalities in power between the actors or parties involved in bargaining. The importance of these recommendations to nurses should not be underestimated; in many countries in the Region, nurses' terms and working conditions still fall short of the minimum level agreed by governments.

EDUCATION

Education is vital in developing excellence in nursing. It faces the tremendous and perennial challenge of keeping pace with changes in practice, a challenge that is all the greater in countries where financial resources for education are restricted, learning materials are few, and there is chronic underinvestment in educating teachers.

Nurses have long recognized the need for fundamental change in their education systems, and have struggled long and hard to move the preparation of practitioners beyond the vocational or apprenticeship models. The participants at the Vienna Conference *(1)* recommended:

> All basic programmes of nursing education should be restructured, reoriented and strengthened, in order to produce generalist nurses able to function in both hospital and community. All specialist knowledge and skills subsequently acquired should be built on this foundation. Nursing education should include ample experience outside the hospital. Candidates for nursing education should have completed a full secondary education (which may vary from country to country) and have qualifications for ad-

mission that are equivalent to those required by a university or other institute of higher education. The directors of schools of nursing or departments of nursing education, and teachers and supervisors of nursing programmes, must all be nurses.

Legal obligations in respect of nursing education have existed since 1977 in the EU countries. For general nurses, the EC directives require a full-time training of three years covering at least 4600 hours of theoretical and practical instruction, after a general primary and secondary education of at least ten years' duration. The directives also give guidance on the theory and practice elements to be incorporated into the curriculum. Almost 20 years after the issuing of these directives, however, not all EU countries are yet able or willing to comply. In 1994, the CE health committee, advised by a working party on the role and education of nurses, produced further guidance on the implementation of education systems based on the new and changing role of nurses in European societies *(25)*.

Reforms of health systems to meet the changing needs of the population and the goals of the WHO strategy for health for all imply many changes for nursing education. World Health Assembly resolution WHA47.9 *(26)* urged Member States "to give priority to assessing and improving the quality of basic and continuing nursing and midwifery education". There is good evidence that nurses themselves soon rose to this challenge, so the problem was less one of persuading the profession than of persuading governments and other decision-makers that investing in nursing education was investing in health. Some improvements in education have already been achieved and, while the consequences are not always immediately evident in practice, they are among the most important recent developments in nursing.

Innovative approaches to curriculum planning and course delivery in nursing education should be supported at the highest levels, so that programmes are *(20)*:

- based on the most recent assessment of a country's health needs and the need for nursing services;
- problem-based, to promote skills of critical thinking and problem solving;
- grounded in the philosophy of PHC;
- based on current research in nursing practice;
- culturally appropriate; and
- multidisciplinary, where appropriate, to encourage shared learning and greater understanding between professions.

A recent WHO Study Group *(3)* noted two different models of nursing education. In one, the education of nurses is not simply a matter of professional competence but involves wider questions about women's right to participate in higher education and to reap its benefits. The ultimate goal is to develop nurses' intellectual capabilities as fully as possible, and in the process to enhance the social and career mobility of women whose opportunities might otherwise be restricted. In the second model, nursing education is simply about teaching people to perform a range of specific tasks. The Study Group pointed out tensions between attempting to improve the general education and status of women through nursing education, and finding an affordable means of ensuring that essential nursing tasks are carried out. Current European reforms in nursing education lie somewhere between these two poles, although closer to the first. There is a growing conviction, with some evidence to back it up, that a well educated practitioner provides better value for money, although she or he is more expensive to train and to pay than a nurse trained only to perform tasks.

Many countries are improving basic and continuing nursing education, as shown in a recent WHO study *(5)*. Nursing education is moving from vocational training to university education, with various stages in between. Nurses and midwives are now educated at university level in many countries. The Vienna recommendations *(1)* and the 1995 Expert Committee *(20)* encourage this trend, although the Study Group suggested that there is a case for developing programmes at a variety of educational levels to reflect the need for differing levels of knowledge and skills *(7)*. It said placing basic nursing education in the university might improve the status of nursing and enhance recruitment, but might also encourage élitism and prompt some countries to increase the proportion of unqualified personnel.

The Expert Committee advocated improved opportunities for mature entrants, and the active recruitment of candidates from rural areas and minority cultures. The Study Group noted, however, that, when students leave their rural communities to be educated in a central, specialized school of nursing, many do not return, and those who do often find that their education and exposure to outside influences have resulted in alienation from their own community. Yet small, widely dispersed schools of nursing may lack the resources and equipment to provide a good education.

Finally, the Expert Committee noted that highly educated nurses do not always remain in clinical and public health practice. Inevitably and properly, some become leaders, managers, teachers and researchers.

Many leave clinical work or indeed the profession, however, because of restrictions in the scope of practice and lack of participation in decision-making. Good structures for clinical and public health careers are vital to keep the majority of highly educated nurses in practice.

Basic education

In many CCEE, the existing medically oriented nursing education systems are being thoroughly reformed to meet international guidelines and directives, notably those of WHO and the EC. This requires a huge effort to replace low-level vocational training, which was often part of secondary education, and had a curriculum containing a large proportion of non-nursing subjects. The determination with which nurses are advocating and tackling this change is one of the major achievements of the last few years. General nursing education is already 3–4 years long in most CCEE (Table 7), depending on the number of years of secondary education and level of nurse training, and is gradually moving to the recruitment of entrants who have completed secondary school. Entry requirements to courses in individual CCEE vary widely, however; the minimum age of entry ranges from 14 to 18 (Table 8), and the minimum years of previous secondary education range from 8 to 12 (Table 9). There is a general trend towards raising entry requirements to make them comparable with those of university courses, but some courses, such as those in Croatia and Slovenia, combine secondary education and general nursing training. In some countries, students have to pass an entrance examination and prove physical and mental fitness.

Table 7. Length of general nursing training in the European Region

Length (years)	Country
2.0	Turkey[a]
2.5	NIS[a]
3.0	Austria, Belgium, Germany, Estonia, France, Iceland, Ireland, Italy, Lithuania,[b] Luxembourg, Latvia, Portugal, Romania, Spain, Slovenia,[a] Sweden, United Kingdom[a]
3.5	Finland,[c] Greece, Netherlands,[a] NIS[a]
3.8	Denmark
4.0	Croatia, Finland,[b] Greece, Hungary, Slovenia,[a] Turkey,[a] United Kingdom[a]

[a] Depending on the number of years and/or level of secondary education.

[b] Including mandatory internship of 6 months.

[c] Depending on the nursing specialty chosen at the outset (midwifery education lasts 4.5 years).

Table 8. Minimum age of entry to general nursing training in the European Region

Age (years)	Country
14.0–15.5	Croatia, Czech Republic, NIS,[a] Slovakia, Slovenia,[a] Turkey[a]
16.0	Austria, Italy
17.0	Finland, France, Germany, Ireland, Luxembourg, NIS,[a] Spain
17.5	Netherlands, United Kingdom
18.0	Belgium, Denmark, Greece, Hungary, Iceland, Norway, Poland, Slovenia,[a] Switzerland

[a] Depending on the level of general nursing training.

Table 9. Number of years of primary and secondary education required before entering general nursing education in the European Region

Years of education	Country
8	Croatia, Slovenia[a]
9	Czech Republic, Slovakia, NIS[a]
10	Austria, Denmark, Finland, Italy, Netherlands,[a] Turkey
11	Bulgaria, France, Germany, Luxembourg, Netherlands,[a] NIS[a]
12	Albania, Belgium, Estonia, Finland, Greece, Iceland, Ireland, Israel, Lithuania, Latvia, Norway, Portugal, Spain, Slovenia,[a] United Kingdom

[a] Depending on the level of general nursing training.

Some country examples show the many efforts under way in the CCEE. In Hungary, the 1993 model of nursing education follows EC directives and WHO guidelines. A few programmes last four years, and a further two years' postgraduate study results in a university diploma, designed to produce future leaders in management, research and education. The other new programme, in which most students will be trained, will take place at independent schools of nursing, last three years and focus more on practice. In Poland, a new programme lasting 2.5 years was introduced in 1991 and almost all students follow it. The plan is to offer it to students who have completed their secondary education. It is being evaluated and the findings will be used to draw up a new three-year curriculum. After qualifying, the nurse must undergo 3–6 months of supervision in her or his first hospital post; she or he may not perform nursing duties alone and must work under supervision. The nurse is then assessed by more senior nurses before being permitted to practise independently.

In Romania, general nursing training moved to high schools in 1978, reducing a professional education to a short apprenticeship; the entry requirement was eight years' general education, so trainees were young teenagers. In December 1989, a national nursing task force was established by nursing activists, supported by WHO and the United Nations Children's Fund (UNICEF), and the 41 district schools of nursing reopened in 1990. The task force was officially recognized by the health ministry in 1992, and the following action plan was drawn up:

- developing a three-year programme to meet European standards for the general nurse, with one-year postbasic courses for the priority areas of community nursing, psychiatric nursing, midwifery and social work;
- providing continuing education for those trained before 1978;
- providing a bridging programme for those trained between 1978 and 1992; and
- developing postbasic training for education, management and clinical practice.

A new general nursing curriculum was designed and introduced in some of the reopened district schools of nursing in 1992. Work has begun on the training of trainers and the production of good teaching materials. In very difficult circumstances, progress on nursing education has been surprisingly good. A dispute between the health and education ministries over control of the nursing schools was a major obstacle; they were put under the authority of the education ministry in 1993.

The governments of both the Czech Republic and Slovakia have identified the reorientation of health professionals' education as a priority. The new programmes are based on the philosophy that nursing is an independent profession, and will focus on a biological, psychological and social model of the person, health education and the skills required in PHC, and management and information systems. The age of entry will be raised; a commission will be set up at the health ministry in each country to accredit courses. A council for postgraduate study, with representatives from the health ministry, the universities, the institutes for postgraduate education and professional societies, will oversee the work of the commission.

Education methods vary among the CCEE. In countries such as Albania and Bulgaria, the lecture format is still used in all schools of nursing. Other countries, such as the Czech Republic and Slovakia, report the use of lectures, group work, modelling, case studies using the nursing process, and brainstorming, but such approaches are only just beginning in many countries. All countries lack modern textbooks written in or translated into their languages and applicable to their needs.

Theoretical assessment of students in all the CCEE is by examination. For example, students in Bulgaria are examined at the end of every term, and take a state certification examination at the end of their training. Senior nurses are usually responsible for clinical guidance and assessment. In Croatia, students are required to work in clinical practice for a year on completion of their nursing studies before taking the state examination.

Similar reforms are proceeding more slowly in the NIS. Despite the lack of overall strategies for human resources development, progress is being made in the Baltic states, the Republic of Moldova and the Russian Federation, while nursing leaders in all NIS are discussing the issues and trying to secure high-level support for reform. Nursing education is still usually conducted under medical control as part of the training of middle-level health personnel. The directors of training institutions are doctors, and nurses and feldshers make up only a very small part of the teaching staff. The top fifth of graduates from nursing schools usually move on to train as doctors, so many doctors have worked as nurses. Nursing education is thus seen only as a lower form of medical training, and nursing is not seen as a worthy career in its own right. In all the NIS, students must pass a state examination at the end of the course to gain the right to practise. In Kyrgyzstan and Uzbekistan, students with low marks can start to practise as qualified nurses after two years of practical experience, following a clinical assessment by their teachers. The skills developed include feeding patients, caring for the seriously ill, applying dressings and carrying out procedures.

In most NIS, the old Soviet education system is still intact. Students enter the middle-level training school after 9 years' general education (Table 9) and at only 15 years of age (Table 8), and their first year of study includes both general and nursing education. Some 20% are rejected after the first examination; after a further two years (Table 7) the rest can become general nurses, along with students entering after 11 years of general education. Following the third year, the top 20% continue their studies to qualify as feldshers. In all countries entrants have a health check, and most schools have an entrance examination.

The Soviet model was basically the second model outlined by the WHO Study Group *(7)*: teaching people to perform a specific, fairly narrow range of tasks under medical supervision. The level of knowledge and practical skills obtained in nursing schools is low. In general, curricula in the NIS do not prepare nurses to respond adequately to the health needs of the country. General, non-nursing subjects still take up much of the curriculum. Nurses are said to be educated to provide patient care in curative and preventive health institutions, to perform medical procedures and to prevent and detect disease and promote health, although the focus remains on performing tasks to help doctors. In general, nurses are not aware of the principles of PHC, and the lack of learning materials in their own languages remains a major obstacle.

The Baltic states introduced new training programmes after 1990 consisting of three years' training for general nursing. These programmes include a six-month period of clinical practice before students are granted a grade status and permission to practise. Some problems are reported with nursing assistants who need additional training. The Republic of Moldova is also starting reform. In 1993, an experimental three-year programme was launched comprising a mixture of lectures (45%) and practical training (55%) and a clinical practice module, and including new subjects such as social and human sciences. The programme was designed to conform to international standards, and the new national curriculum drawn up in Romania was used as a model. Attempts are being made to reorient the curriculum towards nursing, including the introduction of nursing theory (especially that of the nurse–scholar Virginia Henderson). Efforts are under way to improve the coordination of clinical and theoretical learning through better contact between colleges and hospitals.

In the Russian Federation, a new system of qualification for middle-level health personnel was introduced in 1992. Three grades of qualification are dependent on passing the relevant examination: second, first and highest. Different grades attract different salaries. The first degree-level programme for student nurses has started at I.M. Sechenov Moscow Medical Academy. A new four-year curriculum was introduced in some progressive nursing schools in 1991, and advanced programmes were introduced in 48 Russian nursing colleges from 1991 to 1993. A new course on prevention was developed, with eight modules covering such topics as health and risk factors, family health and lifestyles. Guidelines were prepared for nurse teachers and seminars held to introduce them to new ideas such as the nursing process.

In the NIS, teaching is didactic, with lecturing as the main method and very little use of student-centred approaches. Methods are gradually being modernized, however; for example, group work using a problem-solving approach has recently been introduced in the new programme in Estonia. In all countries, schools are desperately short of resources and have little equipment or information technology. All lack modern nursing learning materials and textbooks of any kind.

Education infrastructures and curricula differ widely in western Europe. Although strongly influenced by the EC directives on nursing, not all EU countries observe them. The reform of curricula and teaching methods is widespread throughout western countries, including Austria, Finland, France, Iceland, Ireland, Italy, the Netherlands, Switzerland, Turkey and the United Kingdom. In most countries, general nursing training takes place in separate schools of nursing or institutes of higher education; except in Greece, where training still takes place in hospital schools of nursing and technological institutions alongside other health professions. There is a trend towards moving the responsibility for curricula from the health to the education sector. Traditional hospital-based curricula are being reoriented to a research basis and to address health care needs and broad concepts of nursing, in order to provide holistic care of patients or clients in their living and working environments. All countries meet the requirement of roughly three years' training (Table 7). Entry requirements for age (Table 8) and years of general education (Table 9) vary widely. Ireland, Malta and the United Kingdom have additional entry requirements related to achievements and examination results from secondary school. In France, additional entry tests must be taken.

In Iceland, the three-year hospital-based programme was phased out in 1986 and all nursing education now takes place in two universities. The departments of nursing cooperate with many health care agencies: students have the opportunity to gain clinical experience in university hospitals, community health centres, day-care, schools, homes for the elderly and the community. Nursing training in the United Kingdom has been reformed by Project 2000, a new three-year programme with four nursing branches: adult, child, mental health and mental handicap. All students follow the same curriculum for the first 18 months before starting their chosen branch. Courses are based in universities and other institutes of higher education, and no longer in schools of nursing attached to hospitals. Project 2000 emphasizes health and includes experience in the community; students are no longer regarded as integral to the health service labour force, but are supernumerary. In the Netherlands, nursing education is being thoroughly reorganized, while a new training programme in France was established by decree in 1992. Training is provided by schools of nursing run by public hospitals, private hospitals, associations and the national education system. The curriculum aims at producing a practitioner trained in general and psychiatric nursing for practice within and outside the hospital. Nurses are prepared to handle all aspects of nursing: preventive care, curative care, rehabilitation, human relations and health promotion.

The reverse occurred in Finland after a comprehensive reform of secondary education and training in 1987. Education as a generalist nurse ceased to exist at the college level, and basic and specialized education were combined. The students choose their clinical specialty at the outset of their studies: medical–surgical nursing, operating theatre or anaesthesiology nursing, psychiatric nursing, paediatric nursing, midwifery or public health nursing. The term registered nurse is still used for those who graduated before 1987 or specialized after 1987 in a field other than public health nursing.

In Turkey, the diploma and Bachelor's programmes each last four years, and the associate degree programme lasts two years. Graduates from all programmes are registered nurses, hold the same clinical responsibilities and perform the same nursing duties. The Government is trying to reorganize this system, and the national health policy of Turkey includes the reform of nursing training. Discussions are under way to end the diploma programme at the schools of nursing, which is a combination of general education and basic nursing training.

A wide variety of teaching methods and techniques is reported in western Europe, including lecturing and group work, demanding active participation by the students. A modular approach is common. Teaching materials and textbooks are up to date in most countries. The availability of learning materials in both mother tongues and foreign languages (mainly English) is generally adequate, although some countries in southern Europe rely heavily on translating foreign texts and journals. Information technology is being introduced rapidly in all areas of health care and nursing education. Students in all western European countries are assessed by examination throughout the curriculum and by final examination, resulting in the award of a certificate, diploma or degree that entitles the nurse to practise.

Teachers of nursing

Ideally nursing students should be taught by suitably qualified nurses, with doctors and other specialists (such as sociologists, physiologists and psychologists) giving some input in clearly defined areas. This is far from the case in many countries, where doctors hold the senior education positions and nearly all the teaching posts. Nurses recognize the need for nurse teachers to have additional training in education and advanced nursing, and are slowly working towards the goal of an educated workforce of nurses able to direct and participate in the education of nursing students at all levels, from basic to doctorate. Special consideration should be given to new ways of integrating teaching and practice, to ensure that education is relevant to practice and to bring high quality nursing theory and practice from educational settings into the health care system.

Most CCEE report training possibilities for nurse teachers, except Romania; data on Albania and Bulgaria are not available. There is a trend towards better education for nurse teachers and specialists. The professional qualifications of nurse teachers vary, as do the settings and duration of training courses. In Croatia, the Czech Republic, Hungary, Poland and Slovenia, nurse teachers are trained at university level; they teach nursing subjects and other health professionals cover the other areas. In Croatia, for example, doctors teach anatomy, physiology and clinical medicine, psychologists teach psychology, and nurses teach nursing. Clinical teachers who run practical sessions part-time have college-level education. Others with university education – psychology or pedagogy graduates – are full-time lecturers. In Slovenia, the lack of nurses with doctorates creates a problem for higher education courses, because legislation requires that lectures be given by staff holding a doctorate. At present, foreign lecturers are sometimes employed to fill the gap.

In Bulgaria, the teachers are mainly general educators, medical staff and specialist lecturers. One of the aims of nursing education is to give an understanding of allied disciplines so as to enhance collaborative work. The directors of the 41 state nursing schools in Romania are either doctors (31) or teachers of general subjects (10). Many teachers are doctors, but 220 nurse teachers are based in and paid for by the schools, and 300 are based in and paid for by hospitals.

In the NIS, about 95% of the people who teach nurses are doctors with little nursing knowledge. Nurses and feldshers on average make up only 5% of the teaching staff. The directors of training institutions are always doctors. The domination of doctors reinforces the medically oriented curricula. Short postbasic courses in nursing education are available, but there is no diploma. The reform of basic curricula and introduction of new topics, such as PHC or communication skills, highlights the urgent need to train and retrain nurse teachers. Even when a progressive new curriculum is developed, very few teachers can teach it.

In most western European countries, teachers at schools of nursing and universities must be qualified health professionals with clinical and practical experience. Usually they must hold a teaching qualification. In Ireland and the United Kingdom, all new nurse teachers must have a Bachelor's degree; in Israel, all nurse teachers are required to hold a Master's degree. In Portugal, nurse teachers in top posts must hold a doctorate. Universities have educated nurse teachers in Finland since 1985, leading to Master's and doctoral degrees. In Norway, 17% of nurse teachers hold a university degree. Nursing subjects are usually taught by nurses and other subjects by appropriate specialists. Most directors of schools of nursing are nurses. The growth of corporate management ideology, however, has opened the door for professional education administrators to become directors of health care education institutions in, for example, the Netherlands and the United Kingdom.

In Spain, teaching posts at faculties of nursing are won through open competition, with the presentation of a curriculum vitae, a teaching project, a master class on the subject to be taught and a list of published work. There are three kinds of teaching post. A lecturer gives theoretical classes only. A lecturer in health sciences gives clinical teaching in health institutions. The third type is the associate. In Malta, all lecturers on the Bachelor's nursing course are nurse teachers from the United Kingdom; this will gradually change as Maltese lecturers gain degrees and teaching experience.

Professional literature

This is perhaps an appropriate point to survey the professional nursing literature on the European scene. As mentioned, most nurses in western Europe have access to books of reasonable quality, written in their own languages and covering a wide range of topics. Some countries, however, still rely heavily on translations of foreign books. In the CCEE and NIS, the lack of books in mother tongues is a serious issue; those that exist are medical rather than nursing in orientation, and they are difficult to obtain and prohibitively expensive for most nurses. Recent changes in the NIS have exacerbated the difficulties, as traditional distribution networks (often from publishers in Moscow) have dried up and inflation has raised the costs of paper and printing.

Nevertheless, efforts are under way to create a professional nursing literature in the CCEE and NIS. A few countries, such as Romania, the Russian Federation and Slovenia, have recently published their own nursing-oriented textbooks, and many have translated foreign books. To bridge the gap until countries are self-sufficient in this area and to build capacity, WHO is coordinating the LEMON project (see Chapter 6 for more details).

In addition to textbooks, professional journals are an important way of spreading information and ideas. They are often relatively cheap and may provide good professional and political material, attractively presented. They help to form opinion, influence decision-makers and encourage debate. Here, too, the east–west gap is very marked. In 1995, WHO compiled an index of nursing and midwifery journals and those that devote space to nursing and midwifery. The range is vast in western Europe – from scientific research journals in specialized fields and monthly newsletters for professional groups to weekly mass circulation magazines of general interest. WHO's index contains nearly 130 titles and there may well be more; every country has at least one journal and some have 20 or more. The proliferation of journals for specialists is a marked feature of recent years, as is the introduction of journals aimed at an international readership. Most nursing and midwifery associations publish their own journal or newsletter; in some cases, this is the leading journal in the country, as in Denmark, Finland and Iceland. Elsewhere, notably in the United Kingdom, rival journals compete for sales; this is the only country in the world with two large-circulation weekly nursing magazines, read by over 100 000 nurses.

In the CCEE and NIS, the full impact of the beginnings of a free press is just making itself felt in this area. For many years, nurses could only read about nursing occasionally, either in a section of an academic journal aimed at and written by doctors, or in a newspaper for all health workers published by the trade union or health ministry. This is still the case in most NIS, although nurses are beginning to use journals more actively to publicize and debate their ideas. Some nurses have a strong desire to start or relaunch a nursing journal; this happened in the Russian Federation in 1995. Progress has been faster in the CCEE and several countries, such as the Czech Republic, Hungary and Romania, now have their own lively, informative journals or newspapers for nurses. Nurses in Croatia and Slovenia have made special efforts to produce attractive newsletters for their developing networks.

Postbasic nursing education

In the current climate of rapid change, nurses must regularly update their skills and knowledge, and the opportunities to do so must be readily available. This might mean taking a first or higher degree in nursing or a related discipline, or a short course to foster awareness of the latest theories and developments in a chosen field. Self-directed learning is increasingly emphasized, with continuing education being offered in a variety of ways to suit the individual's needs, wishes and circumstances. Basic nursing education is seen as only the beginning of a career-long commitment to professional learning. Mechanisms should be put in place to facilitate this. For example, regulatory systems that require practitioners to register their intention to practise can include the requirement to undertake a refresher course. Alternatively, nurses may be required to keep a portfolio recording their postbasic training. Salaries may be adjusted to reflect postbasic qualifications.

As the functions of and demands on nurses have expanded in the last few decades, the demand for good postbasic nursing education has increased, as has the number of specialized courses and qualifications in many European countries. The current interest in producing nurse specialists, especially in paediatrics, mental health and psychiatry, public health, community care and care of the elderly, proves that many countries are making genuine efforts to meet the health needs of different population groups in accordance with demographic, geographical and epidemiological changes. (In some countries, of course, these fields are regarded not as specialties following general nursing education but as professional nursing disciplines in their own right to which direct entry is or should be permitted. This view is declining on the whole, in favour of a generalist-type model of basic nursing education.)

The availability of postbasic courses differs widely in the CCEE. In some countries, such as the Czech Republic, advanced nursing education is institutionalized and very important for the nurse's career. In other countries, such as Croatia, opportunities for postbasic training are very scarce. Overall, the availability of postbasic courses is increasing, although they still focus mainly on the hospital. Courses in community paediatrics, general community nursing and health visiting are sometimes available. Most countries, however, have no postbasic education in geriatric nursing despite the growing need.

In the Czech Republic and Slovakia, nurses receive further education after they have started working, according to the needs of their posts. Postbasic education is mandatory and has two parts: initial clinical experience and professional seminars. The conclusion of the course takes the form of an individual discussion and an assessment of educational attainment. In both countries, advanced nursing is provided by the institutes for further education of nurses. Courses usually last 1½–2 years, and nurses may specialize in a variety of areas. (After finishing these studies, head nurses can specialize in the organization and management of nursing in another two-year course.) In addition, nurses must undertake a research project to secure the general nurse specialist certificate. A system of voluntary extramural education offers seminars, workshops and the like. All nurses have their own so-called visiting cards containing up-to-date details of their professional qualifications, employment, postbasic training and activities, such as published articles. Postbasic education is increasingly a requirement for senior nursing posts.

Nurses in Poland can specialize in surgical, paediatric, psychiatric, theatre, anaesthesiological and intensive care nursing. A nurse must first work for two years in a health service institution in a chosen field. After the qualifying board agrees, a voivodship doctor authorizes the specialist study. The training takes two years and has theoretical and practical components. It is given by a specialist manager appointed by a voivodship doctor, who must have been employed in that specialty for at least five years. Specialist training is available in health promotion and mental health.

In Hungary, after obtaining a certificate in general nursing, nurses can take a year's training in such areas as obstetric, psychiatric, children's and mental handicap nursing to obtain a first-grade specialist diploma. Nurses with this diploma may attend the Central Training Institute for Qualified Health Workers for a year to qualify as second-grade specialists in areas such as intensive care and operating theatre nursing. Registered nurses in Slovenia can specialize in six fields: psychiatric, intensive care, community, ophthalmological, obstetric and gynaecological nursing.

Romania has only one postbasic nursing centre, the Postbasic Nursing School in Bucharest, which offers programmes of 1–4 weeks. It is expected to play a role in planning postbasic training for the whole country, focusing initially on education, management, and maternal and child health, mental health, psychiatric and community nursing. The Institute for Health Services Management, Bucharest, expressed interest in sharing with the School the management training of chief nurses and public health training for other nurses, but no firm plans have been made. Little in-service training takes place, although by law every unit is responsible for organizing programmes. The Romanian Nurses Association organizes some postbasic training courses and conferences in local centres, and foreign donors offer others ad hoc.

In Albania, Bulgaria and Croatia, the state provides no full postbasic training. Minimal in-service nursing or specialty training is available in Albania, but the needs for specially trained nurses are not met in many areas. In Croatia, the new plans for the reform of nursing education include postbasic courses for nurses in some areas. In Bulgaria, there are plans to commence courses at the Institute of Nursing Education in Sofia. The Ministry of Health has asked the professional nursing association to plan legislation requiring nurses to have regular postbasic training.

In the NIS, all middle-level health personnel are required to take refresher courses every five years – in theory. These are usually organized by a centre for continuing education and in-service training in the capital city. In practice, nurses cannot always fulfil their legal obligation to attend; particularly in rural areas, many people take courses only every 15 years, as reported in Kazakstan, for example. While programmes are usually available on a variety of topics, such as management, anaesthesia, surgery, physical therapy, obstetrics, paediatrics and psychiatry, they focus mainly on providing medical assistance, not nursing expertise. These state-funded programmes usually last 1–4 weeks and focus heavily on the hospital, although there are some courses in community nursing. To enter, nurses must have passed the state examination and have two or three years' practical experience. In addition, hospitals arrange study days, and in recent years donor organizations have organized seminars and conferences in most NIS.

In the Russian Federation, 40 postbasic nursing schools and 50 departments in basic nursing schools provide short continuing education courses. There are more than 100 different programmes, lasting from 2 weeks to 6 months. The number of programmes offered in the central Asian republics ranges from fewer than 10 in Kyrgyzstan to nearly 100 in Kazakstan. Lithuania has 255 postbasic training programmes, lasting from 1 week to 3 months.

In most western European countries, postbasic or continuing education programmes are offered to registered nurses in many specialties and activities, such as paediatrics, mental health and psychiatry, public health, obstetrics, intensive and emergency care, medical imagery and radiotherapy, operating theatre nursing, teaching and management. Geriatric nursing is a relatively new field of specialist training offered in some countries. Postbasic education takes place in separate institutes or in colleges or universities. In-service training is provided in hospitals and health centres. Nurses must usually have two years of clinical experience before they can enrol.

Some examples may offer some additional insight into how postbasic training is legally established and organized within the health care or education sector. Spain has two distinct types: regulated training in specialities and continuing training. The specialities in nursing are defined by decree: obstetric–gynaecological nursing, paediatric nursing, mental health nursing, community health nursing, special care nursing, geriatric nursing and nursing management and administration. The courses lead to diplomas as specialist nurses. The teaching is done in units consisting of a university nursing school and the relevant health service institutions. Courses last two years for midwives and one year for others. Students are paid a salary (about 80% of their full salary) and have a contract. In the public sector, continuing training is financed by the Ministry of Health and Consumer Affairs and the National Health Institute; in addition, funds from the total budgets of health institutions are reserved for continuing education. Other public and private institutions also give courses.

In Germany, two-year in-service training programmes are available in intensive care, psychiatric care, operating theatre nursing, oncology nursing, community care and hygiene. In general, theoretical instruction lasts 240 hours, with 85 weeks' clinical experience. Nurses often attend evening classes to study intensive care, psychiatric care, dialysis, operating theatre nursing, community nursing, and paediatric psychiatry, dialysis and neurology. In addition, nurses and midwives can take courses on ward administration (3 months), management (1–2 years), and education (1–2 years). Open learning courses pioneered by the University of Oldenburg are now available to nurses from six universities.

Nurses in Italy have a legal obligation to take a postbasic education course every five years. Specialist training, which is not mandatory, is provided at schools of nursing and through regional programmes in several fields, of which the following are recognized nationally: leadership (head nurse), paediatrics, anaesthesia and recovery. Postbasic training for public health nurses is available at specialized schools of medicine, public health and social service. There is legal provision for secondment on salary, with or without payment of expenses; for special leave of varying duration; and for other types of release from duty for given periods.

In Norway, one-year postbasic programmes in colleges include public health nursing, midwifery, psychiatric nursing and geriatric nursing. Entrants must be qualified general nurses. In addition, there are in-service courses in intensive care and anaesthesia that last 16–18 months. In Finland, according to the act on health care professionals, personnel are responsible for maintaining and developing their professional skills. Furthermore, employers must create opportunities for personnel to take part in continuing education. Nurses can apply for various courses at different institutions. Adult education departments at health care institutes arrange a variety of studies lasting 6–12 months and covering different themes, as well as shorter courses. Employers, universities, polytechnics, associations and other institutes arrange in-service education. The costs of continuing education are paid by employers, nurses and sometimes the students' local authorities or the state.

Higher education

In many countries, nurses and midwives receive their basic education at university level. While some countries show a trend towards university education for all, others tend to educate a small core of professional nurses and a large number of auxiliary personnel. The move to higher education is therefore subject to various interpretations; in view of the wide differences in local circumstances and needs, educational systems, available resources and other factors, it is difficult to design an educational model that would be appropriate or feasible everywhere. In some cases, training is wholly vocational, controlled by the health sector and takes place in schools of nursing attached or affiliated to hospitals. In others, it may be controlled by and take place in institutions of higher education.

In some CCEE, the former Czechoslovakia, Hungary and Poland, university courses for nurses have been established for many years. Other countries have recently established opportunities for higher education, such as Albania and Slovenia, or are in the planning phase, such as Bulgaria.

University education became available to nurses in Czechoslovakia in 1960. Entry requirements include graduation from a secondary school of nursing, preferably with nursing experience. The studies are interdisciplinary and involve the faculties of philosophy and medicine; the former is responsible for the education of teachers. The nursing curriculum includes psychology and pedagogy. A full-time nursing programme (a five-year Master of Nursing programme and a three-year Bachelor's programme) has been available since 1980. Academic qualification is by thesis and state examination. The programmes are designed mainly for nurse managers and teachers, but offer opportunities for those without previous experience. A few nurses study for doctorates.

In Poland, university nursing education started in 1966 at Lublin. There are now five programmes in the medical academies, and graduates from these courses comprise 1.5% of nurses. The holder of a Master's degree in nursing has equivalent legal status to other professionals with higher education. It is hoped that this will become an essential qualification for nurse managers and teachers. Four medical academies offer degree courses to qualified nurses; the 4-year programmes can be reduced to 2½ years if the nurse has already taken the teacher training course.

In Slovenia, university education opportunities for nurses began in 1993 at the University of Ljubljana, with a Bachelor's programme in health education. A new nursing degree course is being established in Maribor with the support of the WHO collaborating centre for nursing. In Croatia, education is being reformed and nurses are pushing for an academic nursing programme to include the degrees of Bachelor of Science in nursing or PHC, a Master's degree and a doctorate in nursing. Some nurses have degrees in psychology or pedagogy and a few have obtained a Master's degree in public health or social psychology.

In the NIS, only Estonia, Kazakstan, Lithuania and the Russian Federation have recently established university nursing courses offering a Bachelor's or Master's degree. There are no such opportunities elsewhere, although countries such as Belarus and Latvia are planning to introduce university training. In Lithuania, a faculty of nursing was established at Kaunas Medical Academy in 1990. It admits qualified nurses with two years' clinical experience who pass the university entrance examination. The programme lasts 3½ years; graduates are expected to become leaders in government, teaching, management and clinical practice. There are no nurses on the faculty staff and the curriculum does not meet international standards, but good progress is being made. There is a shortage of adequate specialist teachers. In Estonia, nurses have been admitted to Tartu University since 1991. They must have 12 years' general education, 3 years' nursing education and 2 years' practical experience. The first cohort of 20 students graduated in 1994.

In the Russian Federation, a National Council for Higher Nursing Education was established in 1993. In 1995, the first class graduated from the innovative programme at the I.M. Sechenov Medical Academy, Moscow, which offers a full-time degree programme for qualified nurses. The four-year course includes nursing, biological sciences, education methods and some practical experience; general subjects are included to fulfil university requirements. The intention is to prepare nurses for future leadership positions in practice, management and education. In addition, the Medical Academy has started evening courses in management and education. In Kazakstan, the Almaty Medical–Nursing College has begun a new programme of advanced nursing studies. The programme had 250 students in September 1992, and is intended to enable students to take an additional third year to acquire a Bachelor's degree and a fourth year for a Master's. The curriculum has been revised to abolish non-health subjects, provide more care and practical skills, and offer tuition in the English language.

Nursing education is available at the university level in most western European countries. In countries such as Germany, Greece, Malta and Spain, the opportunity for nurses to obtain a Bachelor's or Master's degree, or Ph.D. in their professional field is a very recent development. In Austria and Switzerland, however, nursing studies are rarely or never taught at university level; nurses who wish to study at a higher level must major in an allied subject and take nursing as a minor subject. Entry requirements to university courses vary; in countries such as Belgium, only registered nurses can attend university, while education at university level is open to suitably qualified secondary school leavers and other health care professions in Iceland, the Netherlands, Portugal, Spain and the United Kingdom.

Nursing faculties in universities are usually financed by the ministry responsible for education or science, or its equivalent, as part of the national education infrastructure. Exceptions include Spain, which has a complex public–private mix in ownership of the 98 nursing faculties; 26 belong to the Ministry of Education and Science, 58 to different public institutions, 10 to private institutions and 4 to private universities.

RESEARCH[3]

In all areas of health care, policy and practice are strengthened by the knowledge and evidence acquired systematically through research. Although awareness of the importance of research in nursing has grown throughout the latter half of this century, the amount of substantive research undertaken by the profession throughout Europe remains limited. Where research findings are available, they are not always effectively disseminated and used.

The crucial importance of research becomes ever more apparent as the value and cost–effectiveness of nursing come under increased

[3] This section was written with the assistance of Alison Tierney.

scrutiny in this era of universal health care reform and cost containment. Nationally and internationally, policy-makers, managers and practitioners are grappling with tighter health care budgets, the rationalization of management, decentralization of services from hospitals to PHC, increased accountability to patients or clients, and new health problems and challenges.

The outcomes of health care result from many contributing factors, including individual, cultural, socioeconomic and environmental factors that interact in complex ways. The task for nursing research is:

- to tease out the impact of the nursing contribution to health care;
- to demonstrate the value and cost–effectiveness of nursing practices and policies; and
- to ensure that the care that nurses provide in any setting is firmly based on the best available knowledge and evidence.

Nursing research has been established and is growing, even if slowly, throughout the European Region. In some countries, mainly those with stronger economies and a tradition of scientific endeavour, the nursing profession has steadily amassed, over the past 30 years, expertise and financial support for the development of nursing research. The United Kingdom and some of the Scandinavian countries, for example, now have a sizeable cadre of trained and experienced nurse researchers, a considerable amount of research activity as reflected in published output, increasing success in securing funds for nursing research, and explicit nursing research strategies at the national level.

In 1993, the United Kingdom became the first European country to produce a government-supported national strategy for research in nursing and midwifery. This strategy is an integral part of an overall strategy for research and development for the NHS as a whole: the government devotes considerable funding to the implementation of these strategies. The aim of this ambitious scheme is to promote evidence-based practice in all the health care professions, and to encourage collaboration among academic researchers of all disciplines and between researchers and the providers and purchasers of health care. The introduction of information systems is strongly emphasized to ensure that research findings are disseminated effectively to practitioners.

Of course, compared with many other countries in the Region, the United Kingdom has economic advantages, the benefits of political stability and a long tradition of scientific endeavour. Even so, research in nursing grew slowly and with little initial financial support. The most crucial positive influence was the gradual change in attitude of British nurses during the 1970s and 1980s, as nursing education began to emphasize the importance of critical thinking, and as nurses in practice took more innovative, reflective and evaluative approaches. Such attitudes and approaches can be developed throughout the Region, even when the profession faces a lack of infrastructure, scientific expertise or funds.

Links with education

A crucial condition is the forging of links between nursing and the higher education system. Where nursing research has infiltrated the universities – and this has been the key to the more rapid development of nursing research in north-western Europe – it can develop much faster and in an environment in which research is not only valued but expected. In such an environment, in a nursing or medical faculty, students are introduced to nursing research from the start of their education and, importantly, they learn how to read and critically appraise research reports. Later in the curriculum, they can learn about research design, methods and statistics. Once basic nursing education is established in the university and the staff have gained sufficient expertise in research, access to postgraduate study (Master's and doctoral degrees) can be negotiated. This is the route by which researchers are trained, and universities are at the centre of every discipline's or profession's research infrastructure.

This is not to suggest that nurses outside universities have no role in research or need for education. On the contrary, practising nurses have a crucial role in research, as they and managers are best placed to engineer the utilization of findings in practice, and to identify the issues most in need of investigation. All nurses are research consumers. In addition, practitioners who have acquired sufficient knowledge may want to initiate their own research, or a practising nurse may want to gain some first-hand experience by collaborating with a nurse researcher or a multidisciplinary research team.

Although university education for nurses has been available in western Europe for many years (since the mid-1950s at the University of Edinburgh), it is a much more recent development in most CCEE and NIS. The exceptions include the former Czechoslovakia, where university-based nursing departments were established in the 1960s. The Commission for Nursing Research in the Czech Republic provides funds for small projects. In addition, the universities of Zagreb (in Croatia) and Ljubljana (in Slovenia) have a history of nursing research. Although war has hampered developments in these countries, nursing research activity continues: the WHO collaborating centre for primary health care in Maribor, partnered by the Slovene Chamber of Nurses, began a three-year study in 1993 to examine the contribution of nurses and midwives and the division of labour among all health personnel. The results of this research will guide the national action plan for nursing and provide reasoned arguments for negotiating with health authorities, the Ministry of Health, the universities and health insurance companies. Research of this kind, with its potential to influence health care policy at the national level, is increasingly important in nursing for all the reasons mentioned earlier. Nurses across Europe – and particularly NNAs – are becoming ever more aware of the value of research as a basis for political bargaining and professional development.

Political change has brought the CCEE and NIS to a position to begin to develop research in nursing. There is little development in the NIS as yet. In Estonia and Lithuania, research is planned to be included in the new university nursing programmes. The WHO collaborating centre for primary health care and nursing in Almaty, Kazakstan, has conducted some research on nurses. In the Russian Federation, an important milestone was passed in 1995 when Galina Perfilyeva of the I.M. Sechenov Moscow Medical Academy was awarded the first-ever Russian doctorate in nursing for her dissertation entitled *Nursing in Russia: analysis and forecast*. Students on the courses she leads at the Academy's Faculty of Nursing (now a WHO collaborating centre for nursing and midwifery) are taught about research and encouraged to undertake their own small studies. A few demonstration projects are under way with foreign assistance. For example, Project HOPE is supporting work at the Burns Hospital in Moscow. Projects of this kind, no matter how small, provide the vital beginnings for the establishment and growth of nursing research in any country.

National and international action

Almost all countries in the Region now actively promote the furtherance of research and research-based education in nursing, although at different paces and on different scales. Interest is increasing in international cooperation in nursing research, nursing education and some specialties, such as cancer nursing. Nevertheless, few multinational research projects of any scale have yet been undertaken in Europe. The most notable example remains the WHO Regional Office for Europe's study of people's needs for nursing care *(27)*. This ambitious project, initiated in 1974, involved 11 European countries, 7 WHO collaborating centres, 23 participating units and thousands of nurses on the ground. It was described in the final report as "a major milestone in the history of nursing in Europe". The findings, published in English, French, German and Russian, have influenced practice development in many countries. Perhaps the project's supreme achievement was the sharing of research expertise between countries, and the involvement of countries in which there had been no previous opportunity for research development in nursing.

WHO has continued to foster the development of nursing research guided by the recommendations of the 1988 WHO European Conference on Nursing *(1)*. They urged the appointment of nurse researchers to all national and regional councils dealing with health or related research, including such bodies as the WHO Advisory Committee on Health Research, and called for further action:

> WHO should urge nurses to start community care demonstration projects that provide measurable improvements in care and promote the efficient use of resources in selected communities.
>
> To permit the development of community-oriented nursing practice, education and leadership, nursing research must be part of all fields of practice.
>
> An equitable share of funds should be made available for nursing projects.

ICN has a similarly long-standing commitment, issuing the first guidelines for the development of nursing research in 1985 *(28)*. In 1987, the ICN Council of National Representatives made a statement, reaffirmed at its 1993 meeting *(29)*:

> Nursing research focuses primarily on developing knowledge about nursing and its practice, including the care of persons in health and illness. It is directed toward understanding the fundamental mechanisms that affect the ability of individuals and families to maintain or enhance optimum function and minimize the negative effects of illness.
>
> Nursing research should also be directed toward the outcomes of nursing interventions to assure the quality and cost–effectiveness of nursing care.
>
> Nursing research also emphasizes the generation of knowledge of policies and systems that effectively and efficiently deliver nursing care; the profession and its historical development; ethical guidelines for the delivery of the nursing services; and systems that effectively and efficiently prepare nurses to fulfil the profession's current and future social mandate.
>
> Furthermore, nurses may conduct and/or collaborate in research related to broader issues of health, illness, health services development and management, policy formulation and education.

In 1990, in partnership with the National Center for Nursing Research in the United States, ICN convened a task force on international nursing research; global progress and problems were reviewed, and recommendations for action published *(30)*. Two major themes guided the task force's considerations, and they sum up the key challenges worldwide:

- the need to develop scientific knowledge to underpin nursing practice;
- the need to bridge the gap between nursing practice and research, so that research findings are channelled to practice settings and topics requiring research are identified by nurses in practice settings.

ICN chose nursing research as its theme for International Nurses' Day in 1996. The material and suggestions for action distributed to NNAs around the world were particularly aimed at countries in which nursing research is still in its early stages, specifically to draw attention to the many ways in which NNAs can promote research.

Europe provides excellent demonstrations of the significant and substantial role that NNAs can play in promoting nursing research in countries *(31)*. Some have taken a particular interest from the outset in safeguarding ethical standards, producing helpful ethical guidelines for nurse researchers and so setting sound standards for nursing research. NNAs have also been instrumental in developing a strong base for international cooperation by their active involvement in the Workgroup of European Nurse Researchers (WENR). This was established in 1978 and its members represent all parts of the Region, including almost every ICN-affiliated NNA in Europe. WENR arranges a European nursing research conference every second year, in a different country each time, and the proceedings are published, containing papers by nurses from every corner of Europe.

Contributing to the better dissemination of nursing research is one of WENR's functions. Conferences are important in this regard but, of course, dissemination relies more on written forms of communication, especially publication in journals. In 1995, WENR began to compile a directory of European nursing journals that publish nursing research reports and research-related papers. This directory will inform researchers, nurses, educators and librarians about the sources of nursing research literature throughout Europe, and should encourage more international publishing and reading. While some countries are well supplied with a range of journals in which research material can be found (such as the United Kingdom, with nearly 40 journals), others have very few. Some can publish nursing research only in the national language, which may keep it from entering the international literature.

Better dissemination is just one of many challenges that confront the Region. To encourage future development to be more systematic and strategic than in the past, an Expert Committee on Nursing Research was established in 1993, under the auspices of the CE health committee. The Expert Committee prepared a strategy paper on nursing research for nursing organizations and health ministries throughout Europe *(32)*. It views research as an integral part of nursing, aimed at providing new scientific knowledge that helps to improve the quality of care.

One of the key recommendations is that every country should formulate a national strategy for the coordinated development of research in nursing. Some countries, as mentioned earlier, already have a national strategy for nursing research; planned and coordinated development at national level can achieve much more, more quickly, than uncoordinated ad hoc initiatives. A model strategy has five key considerations:

- the development of structure and organization
- the integration of research and practice
- the establishment of educational opportunities
- the raising of funds and investment of resources
- collaboration between countries.

All countries should be aware of this important document *(32)* and use its recommendations to direct and support their initiatives, as modest or ambitious as their circumstances allow. Some countries may well be ready and have the resources to set up centres of nursing research, to establish research positions in service settings and to ensure that higher education institutions provide research education. Others may need to set more modest short-term goals, such as taking the first steps towards introducing research into at least some nursing curricula and, for practising nurses, concentrating on fostering and rewarding the skills of reflective practice (rather than those required for the doing of research) and the use of published research findings. After all, there is no point in building a cadre of research experts and a strong research infrastructure without first ensuring that the nurses providing care have had the opportunity to develop a positive attitude towards research.

Dissemination and discussion

As described above, communication within the nursing profession and between nurses and other health professionals and the general public is essential not only to disseminate research findings but also to encourage debate on current conditions and innovations in the delivery of nursing care. Two of the most effective ways of spreading information and new ideas on nursing and midwifery are professional journals and messages broadcast on audiovisual media.

As previously described, many European countries have one or more professional nursing journals and in some countries, such as the United Kingdom, the amount of written information is overwhelming. Sometimes nursing education programmes are broadcast on television or radio, and all countries have television and radio programmes or items on health or health care issues. In all the CCEE except Albania, at least one specific nursing or midwifery journal is published. Although nursing journals from other countries are sometimes available, there is no widespread or systematic exchange of written information. Nursing education programmes and health messages are not widely broadcast on television and radio, mainly because of the high costs.

The NIS differ widely in the use of television, radio and written publications to inform nurses of developments. Countries such as Estonia, Latvia and Uzbekistan have monthly nursing journals, and Kyrgyzstan launched a new journal for health workers in 1993. In Kazakstan, the WHO collaborating centre for primary health care and nursing is responsible for a page on health care in the new journal *Ave vitae*, first published in January 1994. Nurses are fully involved in this venture. The centre distributes as much material as possible, but lacks resources such as paper. The Republic of Moldova has no nursing journal, but the Romanian Nurses Association sends copies of its own journal to the Republic Council of Nurses. No nursing journals are known in Lithuania, Tajikistan and Turkmenistan. Many countries are aware of the value of journals but lack money for paper or printing, as well as editorial and publishing skills. Audiovisual media are used to broadcast health messages and discuss nursing issues in only a few countries. In Belarus, for example, daily health promotion radio programmes and twice-weekly broadcasts on television are reported. The Russian Federation and Ukraine use television broadcasts to communicate with health workers and the public, while nurses in Moscow have a regular phone-in radio programme that attracts considerable public interest.

Quality Assurance

WHO regional target 31 *(18)* calls for "structures and processes in all Member States to ensure continuous improvement in the quality of health care and appropriate development and use of health technologies". Quality can be defined as the extent to which actual practice matches the desired outcomes. Nursing has a commitment to integrating theoretical knowledge and practice. This requires the scrutiny of its own performance; as indicated in the section on research, such scrutiny is a growing and welcome trend everywhere in the Region. Nurses are examining problems that reflect a variety of health needs, and questions important to nursing and other disciplines are being asked about health status, the quality of life and the provision of care. New scientific techniques are being used and theoretical understanding is expanding. A wide array of philosophical perspectives from nursing, medicine and the natural and social sciences is being examined, to lay the foundations of nursing science and to guide selection of the most significant questions and the most creative techniques to improve quality. The range of choices is now overwhelming. The many factors that influence quality include: developing and maintaining effective information, evaluation and registration systems; effectively managing human resources; adequately organizing nursing care; ensuring cooperation and coordination among nurses and other health and social care professionals and providers; and providing sufficient education. Previous sections have looked at these issues separately.

In general, the issue of the quality of nursing has gradually gained interest and importance among policy- and decision-makers, the funders and managers of health care, the profession itself and service users. Rising demands and expectations and the high costs of health services are some of the main influences on this trend everywhere in Europe. Health care managers increasingly view the delivery of high-quality nursing services as an important element in improving the performance of the entire system.

One favoured approach to this task is the development and legislative implementation of standards for nursing practice. This is taking place in many European countries, especially in western Europe and the CCEE. Standards can range from voluntary or obligatory ones determined at the national level by ministries or professional associations, to those set by nurses in a particular hospital department or community team. No matter the type and level of standards, setting them is an important step forward, since it can encourage the formulation of patient-centred goals based on a vision of how the ideal service functions. Setting specific standards then enables an assessment of how far they have been achieved and the further problems that need to be overcome, which creates a continuing cycle of achievement, review, and the planning and implementation of innovations. Of course, as all the preceding information indicates, the countries of the European Region vary widely in the quality of nursing, its stages of development, its use of quality assurance methods, and the mix of methods chosen for use in countries, institutions and teams.

All current initiatives in the NIS to improve the quality of nursing concentrate on establishing the prerequisites: up-to-date legislation and regulatory systems, better education and staff development, better working conditions and more efficient health services. Except for some initiatives, mainly in the Baltic states, the NIS have not been able to tackle the introduction of quality assurance methods to nursing practice, although there is some interest in it and an awareness of the need to begin as soon as some of the major reforms are under way. This is due partly to the severe economic crisis in most NIS and partly to the lack of information, skills and understanding among policy-makers and health care and nursing leaders. At the local level, few if any leaders of health care teams are familiar with either quality assurance methods or the skills needed to help a team to use them. This in turn is the result of poor basic education and the lack of continuing education, textbooks and journals.

Similar conditions and situations exist in some CCEE, such as Albania, Bulgaria and Romania. Other countries reveal initiatives and improvements in many areas. In general, policy-makers, nursing associations, and health care and nursing managers in, for example, the Czech Republic, Hungary, Poland and Slovakia are trying to raise the quality of nursing by paying some attention to improved human resource planning, education, teamwork in PHC, and the rationalization and standardization of nursing skills and practice. Progress is piecemeal and patchy, however, and depends very much on the initiative of inspired individuals rather than the commitment of organizations.

Western Europe shows enormous differences in the stages of development of quality assurance in nursing and in the use and mix of methods. Little commitment and few initiatives are reported in some, especially the Mediterranean countries. On the other hand, the commitment of governments and the nursing profession is strong and many innovative projects have been undertaken in a multitude of settings in, for example, the Nordic countries, Israel, the Netherlands and the United Kingdom. By reforming education, legislation, working conditions and other factors, initiatives aim to improve the context and framework in which nurses practise and the quality of practice itself. Most contemporary European societies value high-quality nursing. The issue of measurement, which lies at the heart of quality assurance, is further discussed in Chapter 8 as a key question facing nursing in the years to come.

One indicator of the depth of interest is the establishment of a European Nursing Quality Network (EUROQUAN). It was launched in 1992 to promote high standards of nursing care through the dissemination of research findings and the application of this knowledge in practice. Sixteen countries have joined, all from western Europe (see Table 4–p.35). In addition, WHO has coordinated networks with similar goals, including one for midwifery in the early 1990s and a francophone intercountry network led by the WHO collaborating centre for nursing in Lyon, France, whose aims include exchanging information and developing standards for practice.

Conclusion

This report on nursing in Europe is an attempt to describe and analyse the context and conditions in which the almost 5 million nurses and midwives in the WHO European Region work. By focusing on some key areas of nursing policy and activity, and comparing countries and subregions, it contributes to a better understanding of the many factors influencing the development and practice of nursing. These factors interact with each other and with the traditions and current conditions in society. While this interaction creates different conditions for practice in different countries, the study shows more similarities than differences in nurses' advantages, problems and choices for development. It also shows the magnitude and complexity of the challenge that countries face: to raise the standard of nursing in terms of health outcomes and job satisfaction.

Despite the difficulties of reorienting nursing towards patient-centred PHC, alongside high-quality nursing in hospitals, achievements have been made throughout the Region. All countries are working hard to improve the level of nursing education, regulation and practice. Some, particularly the NIS, are taking the first but essential step: health care planners and nurses are thinking about and discussing possible options for the future. Differences in progress arise from differences in the starting points of countries and in the degree of support from policy-makers. There is by no means a simple east–west divide.

The reform efforts under way in almost all European health care systems provide the nursing profession with new opportunities to prove its cost–effectiveness and its willingness to adopt new responsibilities in both daily practice and the management of nursing services. Nurses should keep on trying to improve the way nursing can be measured in terms of input and outcomes, especially health outcomes. These initiatives should be reinforced by the growing bulk of evidence-based research on the outcomes of nursing practice. Research initiatives will therefore need a strong focus on evaluating established and innovative ways of delivering nursing services, especially in PHC. Nurses must also continue critically to review and evaluate their daily practice, adapt to changing circumstances and needs, and record the process. Nurses everywhere should be encouraged to read and write more about their work, to improve the visibility of nursing and the recognition of its importance. Realizing their potential, however, is not a task that nurses can complete in isolation. Their success will be directly related to how far countries value and support nursing and nurses.

References

1. *European Conference on Nursing. Report on a WHO meeting.* Copenhagen, WHO Regional Office for Europe, 1989.
2. International Council of Nurses. Worldwide survey of nursing issues. *International nursing review*, **42**(4) 125-127 (1995).
3. *Nursing beyond the year 2000. Report of a WHO Study Group.* Geneva, World Health Organization, 1994 (WHO Technical Report Series, No. 842).
4. *International labour conventions and recommendations, 1991–1996.* Geneva, International Labour Office, 1977.
5. *Strengthening nursing and midwifery 1992–95: a progress report.* Geneva, World Health Organization, 1995 (document WHO/HRH/NUR/95.2).
6. *Guidelines for public policy development related to health.* Geneva, International Council of Nurses, 1985.
7. Salvage, J., ed. *Nursing in action. Strengthening nursing and midwifery to support health for all.* Copenhagen, WHO Regional Office for Europe, 1993 (WHO Regional Publications European Series, No. 48).
8. *Handbook of resolutions and decisions of the World Health Assembly and the Executive Board, Vol. III, 3rd ed. (1985–1992).* Geneva, World Health Organization, 1993.
9. *Alma-Ata 1978: primary health care.* Geneva, World Health Organization, 1978 ("Health for All" Series, No. 1).
10. *Guidelines for regulatory changes in nursing education and practice to promote primary health care.* Geneva, World Health Organization, 1988.
11. *Report on the regulation of nurses: a report on the present, a position for the future.* Geneva, International Council of Nurses, 1986.
12. Mörgelin, K. & Schwochert, B. *Pflege in Europa von A bis Z.* Eschborn, Deutscher Berufsverband für Pflegeberufe, 1995.

13. *Papers from the Alberta Association of Registered Nurses health information: nursing components working session.* Edmonton, Alberta Association of Registered Nurses, 1993.
14. KARGER, S. *Principles of legislation for nursing education and practice.* Geneva, International Council of Nurses, 1969.
15. *Code for nurses: ethical concepts applied to nursing.* Geneva, International Council of Nurses, 1973.
16. SAWYER, L.M. Nursing code of ethics: an international comparison. *International nursing review*, **36**(5) 145-148 (1989).
17. *Fourth Meeting of European Government Chief Nurses and Collaborating Centres for Nursing and Midwifery. Report on a WHO meeting.* Copenhagen, WHO Regional Office for Europe, 1995 (document EUR/ICP/NURS 94 03/MT04).
18. *Health for all targets. The health policy for Europe.* Copenhagen, WHO Regional Office for Europe, 1993 (European Health for All Series, No. 4).
19. BRIHAYE, A. *Nurses' pay: a vital factor in health care.* Geneva, International Labour Office, 1994.
20. *Nursing practice. Report of a WHO Expert Committee.* Geneva, World Health Organization, 1996 (WHO Technical Report Series, No. 860).
21. BUTTERWORTH, T. Setting our professional house in order. *In*: Salvage, J., ed. *Nurse practitioners: working for change in primary health care nursing.* London, King's Fund Centre, 1991.
22. HIRSCHFELD, M. ET AL. *Nursing personnel resources; results of a survey on perceptions in ministries of health on nursing shortage, nursing education and quality of care.* Geneva, World Health Organization, 1993 (document WHO/HRH/NUR/93.4).
23. WORLD BANK. *World development report 1993: investing in health.* Oxford, Oxford University Press, 1993.
24. VERSIECK, K. ET AL. *Manpower problems in the nursing/midwifery profession in the EC: summary and policy conclusions.* Leuven, Hoger Instituut voor de Arbeid, 1995.
25. EUROPEAN HEALTH COMMITTEE WORKING PARTY ON THE ROLE AND EDUCATION OF NURSES. *The role and education of nurses.* Strasbourg, Council of Europe, 1994.
26. *Forty-seventh World Health Assembly, Geneva, 2–12 May 1994. Resolutions and decisions. Annexes.* Geneva, World Health Organization, 1994 (WHA47/1994/REC/1).
27. *People's needs for nursing care: a European study.* Copenhagen, WHO Regional Office for Europe, 1986.
28. *Guidelines for nursing research development.* Geneva, International Council of Nurses, 1985.

29. *Resolution on nursing research*. Madrid, Council of Representatives of the ICN, 1993.
30. *Report of an International Taskforce on Nursing Research – 1990.* Geneva, International Council of Nurses, 1992.
31. Abrams, S. Nursing research resource development. Epilogue. *International journal of nursing studies*, **27**(2) 175-177 (1990).
32. European Health Committee. *Nursing research: report and recommendations.* Strasbourg, Council of Europe, 1996 (document).

Part II
Strategies for Action

3

Nursing up to and beyond the year 2000

Jane Robinson & Ruth Elkan

WHO and other organizations have produced much vision and guidance in recent years about the direction that nursing is likely to take in the coming decades. In this chapter we look at recent reports on the future of nursing. Many identify similar issues and concerns. One common theme is the need for nurses to understand the wider socioeconomic context in which they work. As the end of the twentieth century approaches, one can identify the following broad trends that will shape nursing in the next century:

- population growth, resulting in increasing pressure on natural resources;
- increasing numbers of dependent people, as the proportions of the elderly and the very young increase relative to the proportion of people who are economically active;
- the explosion of knowledge and technology; and
- the fluctuating social, economic and ethical climate in many countries in the European Region, which has had a profound influence on health.

Methods of dealing with many health problems are improving, but many countries cannot afford the fruits of increasing knowledge and better technology. Expectations have been raised but cannot always be satisfied, and inequalities in access to health care are likely to increase further. Many countries are characterized by economic recession and growing divisions between rich and poor; some have seen a resurgence of racism and violence.

Some of the consequences of these demographic, economic and political forces are described in more depth. Most of the data come from the latest WHO report on health in Europe *(1)*.

Inequalities in Health in Europe

We suggested above that improved technology for dealing with health problems is not equally available to all, and that the socioeconomic and political climate in many countries militates against the achievement of health gains. Evidence from a range of sources confirms that inequalities in people's health between countries of the WHO European Region not only exist, but are also growing *(1)*.

Mortality rates

The east–west gap in life expectancy opened in the 1960s and has widened in recent years. Life expectancy has steadily increased in the southern, northern and western countries; in the CCEE, however, life expectancy has failed to increase since 1990. Most worryingly, life expectancy in several NIS has dropped to the lowest levels for decades. Similar disparities are apparent in infant and maternal mortality rates. Infant mortality ranges from 5–8 per 1000 live births in most Nordic and western countries to over 40 per 1000 in some central Asian republics. Maternal mortality ranges from zero in small countries, or about 3 deaths per 100 000 live births in Greece, to over 60 in Kyrgyzstan and even more in Turkey. Although maternal mortality has declined overall, there is evidence of increases in some of the CCEE and NIS.

Leading causes of death

The health gap appears in statistics on the three leading causes of death in the European Region. Cardiovascular diseases are the first of these, causing about half of all deaths in the Region. They are the main component of the east–west mortality gap. Cancer is the second leading cause, and is responsible for about 20% of deaths. Falling rates in EU and Nordic countries are accompanied by rising rates in the CCEE and NIS. The diverging trends in cancer mortality are due in part to mortality from lung cancer: higher rates of smoking undoubtedly provide the explanation for increasing rates of lung cancer in eastern countries.

The third leading cause of death is external causes, which include injuries, accidents, poisoning, homicide and suicide. Mortality from these causes is declining in most western countries, but increasing in almost all the CCEE and NIS. The transition to market economies in the latter has brought in its wake increasing social violence, less stringent occupational safety measures and growing psychological stress. These factors, combined with excessive alcohol consumption in some NIS, are reflected in the increase in mortality from external causes of death, particularly homicide.

Armed conflict

In 1992 alone, wars affected at least eight countries in the European Region. Each conflict has resulted in the death of 1000 people or more per year. During 1992 and 1993, armed conflict in the former Yugoslavia killed more than 150 000 people, wounded hundreds of thousands more and displaced close to 4 million.

Issues of public health

About 110 million people in the European Region (12% of the total population, mainly in the eastern countries), still lack access to safe drinking-water. Even more are not served by adequate sewage treatment facilities. Waterborne infections have become a major problem, particularly in the CCEE and NIS. There has been an increase in the incidence of typhoid, cholera and hepatitis A, as well as other gastrointestinal and parasitic diseases, particularly in the central Asian republics and the Russian Federation. For example, 165 cholera cases were registered in Tajikistan in 1993, and a large outbreak (over 1000 cases) occurred in Dagestan in the Russian Federation in 1994. Such findings indicate the need for basic sanitation systems as a high priority in many countries.

The persistence and increase of tuberculosis are also associated with inadequate socioeconomic conditions. It is a problem for the entire Region. There have been 2 million new cases of infection in the Russian Federation and CCEE in the last five years, and 29 000 deaths *(2)*. Tuberculosis notification has also increased in many western European countries. With the current trends towards increases in mass migration, numbers of refugees and poverty in many countries, transmission of the disease is likely to increase.

The number of homeless people in the Region remains substantial – 3 million in the EU alone. Millions more live in shanty towns. The problem is aggravated by the growing number of violent conflicts and political upheavals in many countries, with large-scale migration increasing the numbers of refugees seeking shelter. Economic recession, which affects countries throughout the Region, is pushing more and more people into unemployment, poverty and homelessness. Homeless families face increased health risks from accidents and violence, and from respiratory and infectious diseases *(2)*. Housing is associated with about 60 000 deaths and 50 million cases of injury and disability treated each year. In areas of armed conflict, the disruption of water and electricity supplies has resulted in extreme hardship for millions of people. Furthermore, a third of the Region's population lives in cities with air pollution levels above the WHO guideline limits.

In addition to physical conditions, psychosocial conditions are deteriorating in many places. In many cities, social polarization into affluent and deprived areas is becoming more entrenched. In neighbourhoods with high concentrations of unemployed people, people on low incomes and lone-parent families, local economies are deteriorating. Local services are becoming overloaded and eventually breaking down, and crime and vandalism are increasing. Fear and depression are adding further to the decline of neighbourhoods *(2)*.

Vulnerable population groups

Certain groups in the population are more vulnerable to ill health and premature death than others. Vulnerable groups include women, children, the elderly, the poor, migrants, refugees and displaced people.

Women are, in the main, responsible for caring for the young and the old, yet their health is usually worse than that of men. Although women live longer, they suffer higher rates of chronic illness and disability. In addition, women's economic situation is usually poorer than that of men, which also has important implications for health. Improving women's health is an important goal in itself, but it is also important because women's health affects family health in general.

The elderly are the most vulnerable population group. Their plight is particularly acute in the CCEE and NIS, where they have been the first to suffer from the consequences of economic crisis. Rampant inflation in recent years in the NIS has virtually wiped out elderly people's savings. State pensions are too low to pay the increasing costs of housing, heating and food, while economic crisis has affected state funding of residential institutions for the elderly. International aid has been vital in helping to meet the basic needs of those in residential accommodation.

Migrants and refugees constitute especially vulnerable groups. They are concentrated in urban areas, alongside other socially marginalized people. This has resulted in poor sanitary and living conditions, particularly homelessness and substandard housing. Many migrants and refugees live below the poverty line. Migrants and refugees comprise from 11% to almost 40% of the population in the various CCEE, while the average in the EU is about 15%. They experience not only physical privations but also social and psychological difficulties associated with integration. Cultural differences and language difficulties often reduce the accessibility and acceptability of health services *(3)*.

Summary – the widening gap

The health gap between the CCEE and NIS and the rest of the European Region continues to widen. Inequalities in health are growing, as are disparities in access to the prerequisites for health such as shelter and food. Certain vulnerable groups, particularly the elderly, migrants and refugees, have unacceptably low standards of living and poor health. Economic recession has led to poverty, unemployment and homelessness for increasing numbers of people. In some countries, the restriction of public spending has led to a reduction in the health and support services provided, with the strongest impact on people of lower socioeconomic status.

What Nurses and Midwives Can Do

How can nurses and midwives help to tackle these health problems? The main source of guidance has been WHO, and we therefore concentrate here mainly on WHO reports and recommendations. We also discuss guidance from the World Bank. Before looking at these reports and recommendations, however, one should be aware that much recent work – in particular that of WHO expert committees and study groups – does not mark a radical departure from the past. Much of the thinking and many of the recommendations can be traced as far back as the 1950s. For example, the need identified at the start of this chapter to view nursing in its wider socioeconomic context was already being stressed by the late 1950s. Similarly, since 1950 there has been an emphasis on the process of health needs assessment – on the need to relate the provision of services to the health needs of the population.

The belief that the role of nurses in maintaining health is as important as their role in caring for the sick has been held since the 1950s, as has the view that nurses should care not only for individuals but also for families and communities. The idea of the public health nurse, performing a generalist role within a PHC framework, is certainly not new but has steadily gained acceptance. Many of the issues that dominated discussion about nursing in the 1950s, 1960s and 1970s – including those related to recruitment and retention, education for the public health role, the need to foster management and leadership skills, and the importance of research – are still uppermost in contemporary discussion and debate.

In addition, many recent recommendations have been reiterated over several decades. For example, in 1950 a WHO Expert Committee looked at the issue of providing literature to nurses in the languages of countries where professional literature was almost nonexistent *(4)*. The roots of today's WHO LEMON project can thus be traced back over 40 years.

Recent WHO guidance to nurses

The 1978 Declaration of Alma-Ata *(5)* led to the development of strategies that formalized the need to deliver effective, low-cost health care to local communities through services situated close to where people live and work. The Declaration was followed in 1979 by the launching of the global strategy for health for all by the year 2000. In 1984 the Member States of the European Region adopted 38 regional targets for health for all *(6)*. Subsequent guidance to nurses has addressed the ways in which nursing can work towards the fulfilment of the principles and goals outlined in the Declaration and the targets. Important recent guidance to nursing has resulted from:

- the first WHO European Conference on Nursing, held in Vienna in 1988, at which all Member States of the European Region were represented *(7,8)*;
- a 1992 resolution of the World Health Assembly, which stated the need for developing mechanisms for assessing national nursing needs, national action plans, and better means of monitoring nursing's contribution to health for all *(9)*;
- the 1993 WHO Study Group on Nursing beyond the Year 2000, convened in response to the recommendations of the World Health Assembly *(10)*; and
- the 1995 WHO Expert Committee on Nursing Practice, convened by WHO headquarters *(11)*.

As a follow-up to the 1988 Vienna Conference, the WHO Regional Office for Europe convened a series of meetings of government chief nurses and WHO collaborating centres for nursing and midwifery, with observers from intergovernmental and nongovernmental organizations. The series started in 1989 and continues at the time of writing. The main purpose has been to facilitate discussion between nursing leaders of the implications of the health for all targets in the European Region, and to review progress in meeting these targets. These meetings have resulted in a series of reports *(12–15)* that reaffirm and build on the vision for nursing outlined in the Vienna Declaration *(8)*. The 1994 *(15)* meeting resulted in an important statement and recommendations; statements from the meetings comprise Annexes 1–4.

The underlying themes of the European targets for health for all *(6)* underpin much subsequent guidance to nurses. Six major themes run through the targets.

1. Equity is the essence of health for all. Equity means that policies should aim to raise the living and working conditions of the disadvantaged so that the standards of their physical and social environments are similar to those of more fortunate groups. Equity also implies equal access to health services.
2. The promotion of health and the prevention of disease are important strategic issues in the policy of health for all.
3. People themselves will achieve health for all. This means that the active participation of well informed and motivated people and communities will be fostered, and attempts made to strengthen individual self-esteem, increase self-knowledge and provide social support.
4. Many sectors of society must collaborate to achieve health for all.
5. A harmonious health service system focuses on PHC and adequate referral services and provides affordable, high-quality care. This means meeting the basic health needs of each community through services that are located as close as possible to where people live, are easily accessible, provide high-quality care and involve the community in the management of complementary public, private and voluntary health institutions.
6. Health problems increasingly transcend national frontiers. Strong international cooperation is essential.

All these themes are reflected in subsequent WHO guidance to nurses. The Vienna recommendations underline the importance of PHC, and urge that nursing practice be based on the principles underpinning health for all *(8)*. The recommendations suggest that nursing practice should focus on:

- promoting and maintaining health, and preventing disease;
- involving individuals, families and communities in care and making it possible for them to take more responsibility for their health;
- working actively to reduce inequities in access to health care services and to satisfy the needs of whole populations, especially the underserved;
- extending cooperation between disciplines and sectors of society; and
- ensuring the quality of care and the appropriate use of technology.

Similarly, the goal of the 1995 WHO Expert Committee on Nursing Practice *(11)* was to ensure that nursing practice continued to strive to achieve the principles of PHC. The Committee outlined five principal components of PHC, the origins of which are to be found in the Declaration of Alma-Ata:

a) universal coverage of the population, with care provided according to need
b) promotive, preventive, curative and rehabilitative services
c) effective, culturally acceptable, affordable and manageable services
d) involvement of the community in the development of services so as to promote self-reliance and reduce dependence
e) approaches to health that relate to other sectors that contribute to development.

The context of nursing practice

Nursing does not take place in a political and economic vacuum; it is influenced by its context, as clearly shown in Part I of this book. One objective of the 1995 Expert Committee was to specify the nature and scope of nursing practice in countries at different stages of socioeconomic development.

The Committee saw no direct correlation between the socioeconomic condition of a country and the scope of nursing practice. It noted that nursing is highly developed and provides all the PHC services in some low-income countries and is poorly utilized in others. In some high-income, industrialized countries, nursing has a limited role and nurses receive a poor education; in others, nursing is highly developed *(11)*. Similarly, the socioeconomic condition of a country and the ratio of doctors to nurses seem to have little relationship. Doctors' availability and scope of practice, however, influence those of nurses. For example, the scope of nursing practice can be wide in countries with an undersupply of doctors, and restricted where there is an oversupply. In addition, the method of payment to doctors affects nurses. Where doctors receive a fee for a service, they may undertake the service or procedure themselves. Where there are no such payments, the services may become part of nursing practice.

Core nursing activities

The 1995 Expert Committee stressed that the activities undertaken by nurses are very broad in scope *(11)*. It described the core activities undertaken by nurses in all cultures and societies according to the following six categories.

The first is managing physical and mental health and illness status. This activity involves assessing the health of individuals and communities, detecting ill health, instigating and interpreting investigations, and selecting appropriate interventions, attending throughout to the experience of illness with the patient.

Second, monitoring and ensuring the quality of health care practices involve such responsibilities as self-monitoring, monitoring the effects of interventions, supervising the work of less skilled personnel and consulting with others as appropriate.

Third, organizing and managing the health care system includes setting priorities with individuals and communities to ensure that multiple needs are met, obtaining specialist services as necessary, coping with staff shortages and maintaining a therapeutic team. It also involves promoting intersectoral work in settings such as community clinics and schools. Nursing must influence health strategies and priorities locally and nationally by submitting information at all levels and actively taking part in the planning of health programmes and the allocation of resources.

Fourth, caring and helping involve establishing a climate for healing. Nurses provide comfort to people in distress, support in managing symptoms and help in ensuring the maximum participation of individuals, families and communities in health care planning, treatment and caregiving.

Fifth, teaching about health is an important function of nursing. Nurses must take advantage of people's readiness to learn and provide appropriate information. In addition, nurses should teach self-care, and guide people in caring for their family members.

The sixth activity is managing rapidly changing situations. Nurses must be able to deal with emergencies and crises through the appropriate allocation of resources to meet rapidly changing demands. In some countries, war, civil strife or natural disasters cause sudden and large-scale changes in the environment in which the nurse works. For example, there may be a sudden need to organize health services for a large number of refugees.

Guidance from the World Bank

The World Bank offers a very different concept of the role of the nurse. Its 1993 world development report *(16)* is concerned about the shortage of health care workers, including nurses, and focuses on questions concerning the most cost-effective or cost-efficient use of staff. While the report suggests that nurses can deliver most essential care, their role is that of a technician of limited scope, trained to perform a particular set of tasks that fit into an overall hierarchy of efficient heath services provision *(17)*. The World Bank believes this model will allow for the most cost-effective use of human resources. Thus, nursing should be founded not on a broad base of knowledge and skills but on a narrow base of technical skills in whose use nurses become increasingly specialized. The efficient use of health care resources is represented here by the use of technicians with low-level training, for example surgical technicians trained to carry out simple techniques such as hysterectomies. The World Bank suggests that graduate nurses could perform a similar role.

This model of nursing is the antithesis of that outlined in the Vienna recommendations, with its implication that the nurse should carry out a range of specified tasks based on diagnostic, treatment and evaluative protocols derived from a medical model of health care. It gives an extended role to the nurse, in the sense that low-grade technical tasks are delegated by the doctor. The dangers of pursuing this type of extended nursing role are widely acknowledged. For example, it can limit rather than extend practice, and prevent nurses from fulfilling their potential *(18)*. By contrast, the Vienna recommendations envisage an expanded role in the PHC sector.

The World Bank's view that optimal efficiency can be achieved on the basis of such a narrow role for the nurse is fundamentally flawed. Efficiency can be achieved by deploying low-grade technicians only in very limited circumstances. A low-grade technical assistant (probably not a nurse) may have a place as part of a surgical team; many health care interventions offer no place for such a role. Efficiency cannot be achieved by reducing the work of health care practitioners to a series of technical tasks; rather, optimal efficiency often results from a highly skilled approach, although the skills used can appear nebulous and intangible and are therefore difficult to define and measure. For example, much of nursing attempts to bring about such outcomes as improved social integration of families through increased social support. The skills required to achieve this goal are not as easily measured as those required to perform a hysterectomy. Moreover, it is often difficult to say which of a range of contributions, including those of different types of health care professional and other people, are the most important in bringing about a given outcome *(17,19)*.

The World Bank's narrow focus entails three dangers. First, it fails to acknowledge that reducing the complex and related skills of a range of health care professionals into a hierarchy of technical tasks may preclude the achievement of many health care outcomes. Second, it may result in the pursuit of only the most measurable and demonstrable outcomes, to the neglect of many other beneficial interventions. This is particularly important in relation to nursing, which focuses on prevention and care, both of which are hard to measure *(7)*. Third, it fails to take account of the diversity of different cultures, and the resources available to different peoples to deal with their own problems. The World Bank thus ignores both the inputs that are not a part of the formal health care system and the need to define and measure inputs and outcomes in culturally appropriate ways *(8,16)*.

The relationship between nursing personnel and other health care workers

Both the 1995 WHO Expert Committee and the 1993 WHO Study Group grapple with the question of the relationship between nursing and other health care occupations. The Study Group outlines an extreme possible scenario in which the separation between nursing and medicine will disappear altogether. Nurses, doctors and other health care workers might be replaced by a generic health care workforce made up of people trained to carry out specific tasks for specific care groups *(10)*. The Expert Committee does not go so far but it, too, suggests that the current divisions in knowledge and skills will certainly change and may disappear *(11)*. Its concern is to find a way of balancing the flexibility of nursing with the need for an efficient division of labour. It points out that, although flexibility and diversity are strengths of nursing practice, they may also be a source of conflict among nurses and between them and other health workers. The Committee believes that, to deploy nursing services efficiently and effectively, managers must have a clear description of the educational preparation and practice competences of all nursing personnel, so as to be able to plan an appropriate mix of skills. Rigid boundaries between and within professions, however, can result in restricted practice. Ultimately, the Committee suggests, the roles of all health professionals, including doctors, must become more flexible to be most efficient. The existing divisions in knowledge and skills will certainly undergo great change.

Challenges to Nursing in Pursuing a Health for All Approach

Nursing is very broad in scope, and covers both community and hospital care. Recent guidance emphasizes PHC, and a generalist role for the nurse working as part of a community health care team. This is not new.

Over 20 years ago, the community health nurse was described as "a generalist, capable of functioning in a health team, of communicating with and motivating people, and of working effectively with ... other workers within the community" *(20)*.

Despite the continued commitment to the principles of PHC outlined in the Declaration of Alma-Ata, however, many countries still emphasize the hospital sector at the expense of the community sector. Participants at the 1989 WHO meeting of European nursing leaders noted the scarcity of community services in many countries, with hospitals in many Member States growing in both size and number *(12)*. In 1983, a WHO Expert Committee *(21)* observed:

> It is apparent that in some countries the primary health care approach to health for all by the year 2000 is not well understood by the politicians and population at large, or even by health workers, and the benefits of primary health care may be seen to result from services that are institution-centred and mainly curative in nature.

This observation is perhaps as important today as it was ten years ago. Although health care professionals understand the PHC approach better nowadays, policy-makers and the public at large still need to learn that nursing's most effective contributions to the overall health of the population are based in the community.

Nursing effectiveness and efficiency

Nurses are increasingly being challenged to show that their work is effective – that it succeeds in doing what it sets out to do. They are also challenged to show that their work is cost-effective or cost-efficient – that it provides value for money. A statement made in 1994 by European government chief nurses (Annex 3) lays particular emphasis on effectiveness and efficiency. It urges that the links between nursing inputs and health outcomes be strengthened by increasing the effectiveness and efficiency of nursing practice; the means to use in this task are critical thinking and research, and better collection and use of relevant data for monitoring and evaluation.

Demonstrating effectiveness

The statement suggests that research must play a vital role in demonstrating effectiveness. Nurses must undertake research to ensure that what they do really makes a difference to people's health. Demonstrating effectiveness involves defining what outcomes nursing is striving to achieve, and determining whether nursing inputs and processes are achieving them.

Nurses should therefore adopt an approach that clearly defines outcomes or targets, so that it is possible to evaluate how well nursing interventions meet their goals. The targets for health for all *(6)* provide nurses with a useful starting point for developing their own more detailed targets, and recent work by the Leeds University Institute of Nursing in the United Kingdom contains useful and detailed methodological guidance on indicators for monitoring the nursing contribution to health for all *(19)*.

In summary, the challenge to nurses in future is to focus more explicitly on what outcomes or targets they are attempting to achieve, and to try to ensure that nursing inputs and processes succeed in bringing about these outcomes.

Demonstrating efficiency

While it is widely acknowledged that countries must strive towards the most cost-effective deployment of the nursing labour force if scarce resources are to be used efficiently, there is no agreement on what and what types of nursing intervention produce the best outcomes at the least cost. Here again, research is necessary to discover the answers. Although the World Bank believes that optimal efficiency depends on breaking down the expertise of health care workers into a hierarchy of technical skills, there is little sound research evidence to suggest that this is the case. The challenge to nurses is to demonstrate not only that the work of more highly skilled nurses is more effective but that it can be afforded. We discuss this issue further below.

Effective and efficient nursing: the economic versus the epidemiological approach

Recent guidance to nurses draws on both epidemiological and economic principles. There are inherent tensions and conflicts, however, between economic and epidemiological approaches to questions of effectiveness and efficiency.

Most of the recent guidance to nurses adopts a predominantly epidemiological approach, which stresses that nursing interventions must be geared towards meeting the health needs of the population. The first task is therefore to identify and quantify the population's health needs, and then to attempt to meet those needs in an appropriate way. Economists, on the other hand, believe that meeting all the health needs of the population is impossible. For them, determining the health needs of the population is not the most important initial question; rather, they ask how scarce resources can best be used to bring about maximum health gain. They argue that, if the ultimate goal is to bring about maximum health gain, the way to do this is not to measure the total burden of health needs but to examine the costs of different interventions in relation to the amount of health gain, or benefit, they produce. The starting point for economists is thus the resources available, not the health needs of the population *(22)*.

While much recent guidance to nurses acknowledges the importance of economic considerations, it emphasizes the effectiveness of nursing interventions in meeting health needs, rather than whether these interventions are justified in financial terms. Nurses must face the potential conflict between the two approaches, and grapple not only with epidemiological questions about the effectiveness of their work in meeting needs but also with economic questions about whether interventions known to be effective can be justified if they consume a large share of resources. Nurses will have to recognize that, no matter how effectively they work, a point will come at which greater effectiveness may have to be sacrificed because it cannot be afforded. Since no country can afford to offer all its citizens every possible effective nursing intervention, the need to set priorities is inescapable.

Economists stress the need to set priorities. They argue that, since resources are finite, the choice to use them in one way entails giving up the chance to use them in another way: an opportunity cost. In other words, if nursing resources are used to implement a particular effective intervention, they are not available to implement another that may be equally or more effective. In future, nurses must pay greater attention to opportunity costs and priority setting. They must be involved in making explicit choices between implementing one intervention at the expense of another.

Equity in the delivery of health care

The economic versus the epidemiological approach

There are also tensions between economic and epidemiological approaches to questions concerning equity. We showed above that inequalities in health and the use of health services are increasing in a number of countries *(1)*. Such findings have kept questions of equity at the forefront of WHO's agenda. From an epidemiological perspective, the most appropriate response to such findings is to attempt to redress these inequalities by targeting resources to the people whose needs are greatest. This epidemiological approach is evident in all recent guidance from WHO. Equity is a founding principle of health for all *(6)*.

Equity is also reflected in subsequent guidance to nurses. For example, the Vienna Declaration *(8)* states: "The persisting inequalities in people's health status, both between and within countries of the WHO

European Region, are politically, socially, economically and professionally unacceptable and are therefore of common concern to all nurses". The accompanying recommendations urge that nurses base their practice on the principle of equity, and that they aim to ensure equal access to services for all groups, especially those who currently underuse health services.

As the report of the Vienna Conference *(8)* points out, however, the pursuit of equity may result in a loss of efficiency. Although channelling resources to those whose need is greatest is an equitable solution to the problem of inequalities, these people may provide the least opportunity for health gains. Their poverty, vulnerability or marginal status may render them least able to take advantage of the health education and other services provided by nurses. Greater efficiency – that is, greater health gain for society as a whole – is likely to result from channelling resources to the people best placed to take advantage of nursing services. Services that are both equitable and efficient are rare; inevitably, trade-offs must be made between the two.

Many nurses dislike the idea that considerations of economic costs must temper the pursuit of equity. Nevertheless, nurses must recognize that the pursuit of equity can be costly, and grapple with questions concerning the relative weights to be attached to a fair and equitable distribution of resources, and an efficient use of resources that maximizes health gains to society as a whole, not to one small section of it. In conclusion, nurses must have some knowledge of both epidemiology and economics if they are to develop a critical understanding of many of today's most pressing problems.

Consumer involvement

One of the main themes running through the policy for health for all and WHO guidance to nurses is the belief that people themselves determine their own health: people themselves will achieve health for all. Well informed and motivated people and communities must participate actively in setting priorities, and in making and carrying out decisions *(6)*. In keeping with this approach, the Vienna recommendations *(8)* stress that nursing practice should be based on the principle of involving individuals, families and communities in care and making it possible for them to take more responsibility for their health.

Current policy statements and guidance to nurses thus reflect the belief that in the next century individuals, families and communities will play an increasingly important role in determining and meeting their own health needs. The roles of nurses and other health care providers are therefore likely to change as people take more responsibility for their own and their families' health *(7)*:

> In the future, people will be involved in developing their own health plans, and nurses will work with them instead of doing things for them. Decision-making will pass to the people. The nurse will be a resource person, working with colleagues from a variety of professions and disciplines in the community (rather than solely with a team of health professionals).

Nurses' role as information givers, enablers and facilitators to both individuals and communities will thus increase in importance. Furthermore, the growth in the proportion of elderly people, coupled with the decline in state-funded institutional care for a number of dependent groups – including the elderly, the mentally ill and others – means that informal care givers will provide an increasing proportion of care. These care givers may need to be taught some basic skills and knowledge *(10,11)*. As the formal and informal sectors more equally share the burden of care for many chronically sick or disabled people, the traditional distinction between the two types of care is likely to become less important. The distinction between the role of nurses and those of other care professionals will also lose importance as they collaborate more closely to meet the range of people's health and social needs *(22)*.

The shift towards greater consumer involvement in the provision of health care has many positive elements, but it also contains dangers. It could lead to greater inequalities and inequities between the richer and poorer sections of society if the consumers whose circumstances make it easier for them to take a greater responsibility for their own health are also able to take greater advantage of the education, support and services provided by health professionals. The aim of fostering greater consumer involvement should not be pursued at the expense of the pursuit of equity.

References

1. *Health in Europe*. Copenhagen, WHO Regional Office for Europe, 1994 (WHO Regional Publications, European Series, No. 56).
2. Whitehead, M. *Health, housing and human settlements*. Copenhagen, WHO Regional Office for Europe, 1994 (document EUR/ICP/HSC 419/B4.2).
3. *Demographic trends in the European Region*. Copenhagen, WHO Regional Office for Europe, 1988 (WHO Regional Publications, European Series, No. 17).

4. *Expert Committee on Nursing. Report on the first session.* Geneva, World Health Organization, 1950 (WHO Technical Report Series, No. 24).
5. *Alma-Ata 1978: primary health care.* Geneva, World Health Organization, 1978 ("Health for All Series", No. 1).
6. *Health for all targets. The health policy for Europe.* Copenhagen, WHO Regional Office for Europe, 1993 (European Health for All Series, No. 4).
7. Salvage, J., ed. *Nursing in action. Strengthening nursing and midwifery to support health for all.* Copenhagen, WHO Regional Office for Europe, 1993 (WHO Regional Publications, European Series, No. 48).
8. *European Conference on Nursing. Report on a WHO meeting.* Copenhagen, WHO Regional Office for Europe, 1989.
9. *Handbook of resolutions and decisions of the World Health Assembly and the Executive Board, Vol. III, 3rd ed. (1985–1992).* Geneva, World Health Organization, 1993.
10. *Nursing beyond the year 2000. Report of a WHO Study Group.* Geneva, World Health Organization, 1994 (WHO Technical Report Series, No. 842).
11. *Nursing practice. Report of a WHO Expert Committee.* Geneva, World Health Organization, 1996 (WHO Technical Report Series, No. 860).
12. *First Meeting of Government Chief Nursing Officers and Collaborating Centres on Implications of the HFA Targets for Nursing/Midwifery.* Copenhagen, WHO Regional Office for Europe, 1989 (document EUR/ICP/HSR 334).
13. *Nursing leaders in action. Second Meeting of Chief Nurses, WHO Nursing Collaboration Centres and Nursing Organizations of Europe.* Copenhagen, WHO Regional Office for Europe, 1991 (document EUR/ICP/HSR 347).
14. *Nursing leaders in action. Report of the Third WHO Meeting of European Government Chief Nurses.* Copenhagen, WHO Regional Office for Europe, 1992 (document EUR/ICP/HRH 301A).
15. *Fourth Meeting of European Government Chief Nurses and Collaborating Centres for Nursing and Midwifery. Report on a WHO meeting.* Copenhagen, WHO Regional Office for Europe, 1995 (document EUR/ICP/NURS 94 03/MT04).
16. World Bank. *World development report 1993: investing in health.* Oxford, Oxford University Press, 1993.
17. Robinson, J.J.A. *Reorienting health care for health gain through human resource development: an analysis based on a reading of the World Bank development reports.* Copenhagen, WHO Regional Office for Europe, 1994 (document EUR/ICP/HSC 419/D3.2).

18. *The scope of professional practice: a UKCC position statement.* London, United Kingdom Central Council for Nursing, Midwifery and Health Visiting, 1992.
19. *Indicators for monitoring the nursing contribution to health for all.* Leeds, Institute of Nursing, University of Leeds, 1994.
20. *Community health nursing. Report of a WHO Expert Committee.* Geneva, World Health Organization, 1974 (WHO Technical Report Series, No. 558).
21. *Education and training of nurse teachers and managers with special regard to primary health care. Report of a WHO Expert Committee.* Geneva, World Health Organization, 1984 (WHO Technical Report Series, No. 708).
22. ROBINSON, J. & ELKAN, R. *Health needs assessment: theory and practice.* Edinburgh, Churchill Livingstone, 1996.

4

National action plans for nursing and midwifery

Felicity Leenders & Jane Salvage

Why does nursing, while recognized as one of the most important functions in any health care system, remain undervalued and underdeveloped? Evidence from around the world suggests that the failure to tap the full potential of nursing is often linked with inadequate or nonexistent policy formulation, strongly associated with lack of leadership. Many countries do not have adequate policies and programmes to ensure appropriate, cost-effective staff performance. Worse, recent surveys illustrate a range of crippling problems, including shortages of adequately trained nurses, high turnover, poor deployment and inappropriate skill mixes. These are often exacerbated by relatively low pay and poor working conditions *(1)*.

Partly as a consequence of these intractable problems, interest is growing in the need to adopt a more strategic approach to nursing. For the last two decades, health care systems globally have changed profoundly; it is evident that nursing should have a major role in health care. As long ago as 1975, the WHO Regional Office for Europe called for the profession to be organized so as to provide not only for continuing and immediate services as at present, but for research and study that would advance both the knowledge and technology of care. The Regional Office worked towards that goal by stimulating debate throughout the Region on what the role of the nurse should be in future and how that vision could become reality. The first stage culminated in 1988 with the first WHO European Conference on Nursing *(2)*: the Vienna Declaration and recommendations that it produced contain a vision and a strategy for nursing in the whole Region *(3)*. Recommendation 8 states that nursing should be included as one of the essential elements of national health plans, based on the regional strategy for health for all, and that nurses should take part in the debate on health policy *(2)*.

WHY MAKE A NATIONAL ACTION PLAN FOR NURSING?

Work on nursing policy and strategy is under way in all parts of the world. Some countries and regions have already produced strategies for nursing, and others are preparing them. Examples include Argentina, Bahrain, Bangladesh, Bolivia, Botswana, Chile, Croatia, the Czech Republic, Denmark, Ecuador, England, France, Greece, Hungary, Kazakstan, Kyrgyzstan, Latvia, Lesotho, Lithuania, the Netherlands, Nicaragua, Northern Ireland, Paraguay, Poland, Scotland, Slovenia, Sweden, Tonga, Turkey, the United Republic of Tanzania, Wales and Zambia. Similar developments are beginning to flourish at the local level. In health centres and hospitals, nursing teams are producing their own mission statements and plans. Whether these are called strategies, policy statements or action plans, they follow the same basic principle – the need to formulate and pursue specific targets for improvement: to know what you want and how to get it, in order to increase your effectiveness.

Nurses are well placed to be agents of change in the health care system and in society as a whole; knowledge and skills in managing change will make them more effective in their role. Thoughtful planning for change through a collective approach and a programme of managerial and educational support are likely to ensure meaningful shifts in attitude and behaviour. In working towards the goal of health for all, nurses need a strategy based on local clinical epidemiology, target setting, and the use of indicators and evaluation based on the comparison of outcomes with other groups and/or over time. Such an approach allows for interactive, flexible, systematic, long-term development.

When they get together to develop policies, nurses are sometimes accused of isolating themselves. This seems odd, as nobody issues similar challenges to doctors or politicians. Perhaps the accusation is partly attributable to stereotyping of or misconceptions about nurses; many people do not yet understand that nurses want to act not simply as pairs of hands but as intelligent thinkers and leaders. Every group that sees itself as having a distinct role in or contribution to health care wishes to create its own vision and plans, whether it comprises nurses, doctors, politicians, citizens or others. Each has legitimate perspectives and concerns, and conducting an internal debate helps to clarify a group's contribution and create a greater sense of purpose. What is crucially important is the need to establish excellent channels of communication between all such groups, to ensure that their policy-making is an interactive process. The work of each group should both inform and be informed by that of the others, and all groups should do this work against the backdrop of an overarching debate about how a country can improve its people's health.

The growing emphasis on nursing policy is closely tied to another trend: an interest in leadership. Nurses and midwives are realizing that they need good leaders to ensure the maximum contribution of their profession to health care and the full recognition of its value. As a workforce mainly composed of women with their attention fixed firmly on the needs of their patients, most nurses did not traditionally see any need to have strong nurse leaders among a country's top health policy-makers and managers. Today, however, they see that care – the essence of nursing – tends to be ignored, undervalued and underresourced unless nurses' opinions and perspectives are articulated and advocated at the highest levels. Without such advocacy, care will continue to be regarded as a simple, basic task, not as what it really is – a complex and difficult job requiring skill and intelligence as well as compassion.

The World Health Assembly recognized the need to improve nursing leadership in 1992. Resolution WHA45.5 *(4)* urged Member States "to strengthen managerial and leadership capabilities and reinforce the positions of nursing and midwifery personnel at all levels … including health ministries" and "to ensure that the contribution of nursing and midwifery is reflected in health policies". The Health Assembly requested WHO to establish a group to advise on "assisting countries with the development of national action plans for nursing and midwifery …". This work was to be taken forward by the new WHO Global Advisory Group on Nursing and Midwifery, set up as requested by the Health Assembly. At its second meeting, held in Geneva in 1993, the Group discussed the issue at length; the meeting report *(5)* reproduced as an annex a guidance document from the Regional Office for Europe on national action plans for nursing *(6)*.

Active support for the development of national action plans came from the highest level of WHO. The WHO Director-General wrote to all health ministers worldwide in May 1994, encouraging them to make use of the guidance issued by the WHO Regional Office for Europe and endorsing the recommendation that countries should develop their own plans. He commented that action plans for nursing and midwifery clearly need to be developed in relation to other segments of the health workforce. It would be opportune to embark on a wider analysis of the total health workforce; this would allow modifications that ensure that action plans are balanced and optimally productive and cost-effective.

Activities to provide assistance in developing these plans were already under way in the European Region, as requested at WHO meetings of government chief nurses and other nursing leaders. The First Meeting of Government Chief Nurses and Collaborating Centres *(7),* held in 1989, had called for recognition of "the vital necessity of involving nurse leaders in the formulation and implementation of national health policies and plans" and for "the creation of national managerial positions which permit nurses to make this contribution". The Nursing and Midwifery unit of the Regional Office began to coordinate collaborative programmes to enable countries to develop national action plans for nursing, and to promote the creation of leadership positions. Few countries had such plans, although some had policies or plans on specific aspects of nursing development such as education or legislation. Some had policies and plans that had not been set down in documents available to the public. Perhaps surprisingly, this was true even of wealthy countries where nursing was highly developed. All countries in the European Region faced a major challenge.

These issues were debated extensively at subsequent pan-European meetings of government chief nurses. In 1994, the Fourth Meeting of European Government Chief Nurses and Collaborating Centres for Nursing and Midwifery *(8)* decided that developing national action plans for nursing was a major task that had to be tackled to secure "the necessary commitment and resources for nursing development for better health". It urged WHO to continue providing help in the development of the plans.

As instructed by its Member States, the Regional Office is making a major effort to support the CCEE and NIS. The Nursing and Midwifery unit began to forge closer links with these countries during the early 1990s, focusing on meetings with their nursing and midwifery leaders. The first WHO meeting of government chief nurses from the NIS was held in Kazakstan in 1993 *(9)*. The participants discussed the policy and leadership issues and concluded that: "Each country should develop a national action plan for nursing, as recommended by the 1992 World Health Assembly. This plan should be endorsed and actively supported by ministries of health". The need for national action plans was reaffirmed at the second meeting of NIS government chief nurses, held in Kyrgyzstan in 1994 *(10)*; the participants recommended that countries should "work on the development of a national action plan for nursing as part of national health policy". The third meeting of this network was held in Stockholm in 1995 and attended by leaders from all the countries that comprised the former USSR. The leaders exchanged information on the progress their countries were making in developing the plans *(11).*

Many nursing leaders in the CCEE and NIS have been quick to understand the rationale for national action plans and to begin work on them. They see that a strategic approach is particularly important at this point in nursing's development. Their countries are undergoing momentous changes that create a confusing mixture of opportunities and dangers. People are questioning traditional values, including assumptions about health care and the role of the state as the protector of the poor and the oppressed. Health care systems are being reformed, under strong financial and ideological pressure, with an emphasis on new thinking and new roles. Nurses, like all other health professionals, cannot expect that their roles and relationships will continue unchanged. Increasingly, too, they will have to demonstrate their value and effectiveness to the people who control the budgets. Those health professions with a clear sense of their hopes and directions are more likely to survive and prosper.

Another major attraction of national action plans for the CCEE and NIS is that they provide a framework that the countries can use to establish their own priorities. This is especially important for countries that currently rely heavily on donations and international bank loans to fund changes in health care. Without a clear sense of priorities based on local needs and wishes, these countries are in danger of accepting all and any offers of help, whether or not the help is really what is wanted, and of having inappropriate foreign models of care imposed upon them. The NIS government chief nurses debated this topic at the 1995 meeting *(11)*, summarizing their views as follows:

> We acknowledge the value of external help from WHO and other agencies and governments in this change process. However, we wish to emphasize that such help should be led by us and our countries, working in partnership with these helpers. This requires a major shift away from market/provider/professionally-led initiatives and systems which foster dependence, towards needs-led ones based on mutuality. This echoes the spirit of [health for all]. It also reflects both the need to reorient health care systems away from narrow professional concerns towards those of society, and the current efforts to develop nurse–patient relationships which place the client at the centre of our concerns.

Armed with a national plan, the nursing leader is in a much better position to tell donors and outside project partners what she or he wants and to be sure that the help is effective.

In addition, experience to date demonstrates that national action plans for nursing provide a logical framework for collaboration between the Regional Office and the European Member States. The Nursing and Midwifery unit and nursing leaders may collaborate on drawing up a plan, and then jointly develop programmes to focus on specific parts of the plan, such as the reform of basic nursing education, management and leadership development, or participation in the LEMON project (see Chapter 6). These programmes are individually tailored to the particular traditions, strengths and development needs of each country.

What is a National Action Plan for Nursing?

Every country has its own traditions, strengths, leadership styles and priorities, so national action plans for nursing are not intended to provide an international blueprint. Furthermore, the global trend towards decentralization and the strengthening of local health systems underlines the role of national plans in giving general guidance and emphasizing expected outcomes, leaving the details of how the outcomes should be achieved to be decided at the regional and local levels. Nevertheless, nursing leaders everywhere share many of the same problems and challenges, so the discussion of policy and planning issues in international meetings and bilateral exchanges can help to deepen understanding, put the issues in context and promote new ideas. Indeed, such exchange is also fruitful at the regional and global levels. For example, the WHO Regional Office for the Western Pacific has recently drafted a manual on policy development that contains a great deal of material valuable for nursing leaders in Europe *(12)*.

A national action plan for nursing is part of a continuing process of describing visions, choosing priorities, winning widespread support, taking action and evaluating the outcome. Each stage of the process requires careful attention; this chapter focuses mainly on the initial steps. The plan is not produced in an office by a few administrators, but is the fruit of much debate among many interested people. Without such debate and commitment building, no paper exercise – however sensible and coherent – has any chance of long-term success.

As suggested above, a national action plan can have many different names but always has certain key features: an analysis of the current situation, a description of a vision for the future and indications of the steps to be taken to turn the vision into reality. The plan should be closely linked to the overall national policy for health and health services. Ideally, the plan for nursing is one of a comprehensive series of interlinked plans designed to improve health in specific settings, such as PHC services, acute services, schools or workplaces, or to tackle specific health problems. It is also a key component of the national strategy on human resources for health. In countries where such strategies are not well developed, nursing can help to lead the way by demonstrating its own commitment to the strategic approach, and encouraging others to adopt a similar process.

Some countries regard nursing and midwifery as one profession, while others have separate regulatory, educational and professional bodies for the two occupations. In using the term national action plans for nursing, we do not imply any assumptions about nursing's relationship to midwifery. The need for leaders to promote a strategic approach to development is just as crucial for midwifery as for nursing, but whether this is done jointly or separately is a matter for each country to decide. Either way, it is in the interest of both groups to define their goals and to work together on many areas of mutual concern. The same point applies to other occupational groups that are regarded by some countries as part of the nursing workforce, such as feldshers, physiotherapists and community health workers. The principles of strategic planning are applicable across the board.

The most visible product of the national strategic planning process for nursing is a brief written document, usually endorsed by health policy-makers and leaders at the highest level, such as the health minister. This document should contain a vision of nursing for the future, perhaps for the next 5–10 years, describing how nurses can help people to improve their health, cope with their illness or disability and die with dignity. It sets out specific goals that will help to make that vision a reality, and analyses the current obstacles to be overcome. It might also indicate the next steps to be taken to reach those goals, while respecting local autonomy. This document may be widely circulated among the public, policy-makers and professionals, and its messages reinforced through other means such as discussion and debate in the mass media and other fora.

Why Does a Country Need a National Action Plan for Nursing?

A continuing planning cycle – producing a national action plan, taking steps to implement it and reviewing what has happened – assists the development of nursing in many ways. Some of these have already been discussed above. Ten advantages are summarized here.

1. A national action plan can ensure the orientation of nursing towards health. It reinforces the goal of nursing as promoting improvements in the health of individuals and populations, with an emphasis on results or health outcomes.

2. A national action plan can optimize nursing's contribution to health and health care by providing a focus for mobilizing all available nursing resources to achieve the best possible results and the best value for money.
3. A plan can build and maintain a vision for nursing. When immersed in the details and difficulties of everyday work, nurses can easily neglect their visions or regard them as irrelevant idealism. A vision of where they want to go, especially when they share it with others, is an essential source of nourishment and inspiration.
4. A national action plan can give a clearer sense of direction. The day-to-day challenges of work often make nurses feel overwhelmed and confused. They can cope more easily with this feeling if they keep hold of an overall sense of where they are going.
5. A plan can make nursing's achievements more visible. Many of the finest achievements of nursing are warmly appreciated by patients and clients, but are not acknowledged in medical textbooks, conferences or influential discussions. The visibility given by the plan can lead to greater recognition and therefore greater equity in health systems.
6. A national action plan can spur nurses and their supporters to be more active. The process of strategic planning helps to uncover or inspire unexpected new coalitions, which can then work together to improve health care.
7. A plan can coordinate current nursing activities. The planning process helps nurses to identify what projects and innovations are already under way, to link them more closely together, to strengthen them and to create clear frameworks for future development.
8. A national action plan can create closer links between policy and practice. Policy-making is too often remote from the people responsible for implementation. A planning process involving service users, practitioners and educators, as well as policy-makers, helps to reduce the usual damaging gaps between thinking and action, data and perceptions, policy and operations, planning and implementation, and experts and workers.
9. Nursing is more likely to win support from the people, policy-makers and other professionals if it can state clearly where it is going and what it hopes to achieve. Such support includes commitment and respect as well as money.
10. A national action plan can help nursing control its own work and future. Nurses have traditionally had little control over their destiny, being seen only as servants of another profession. A strategic plan is the starting point for becoming equal partners in health care work and in relationships with other professionals and the public. This in turn will help nursing to play its full part in ensuring health gain.

How Can Nurses Develop a National Action Plan?

When people think about developing a strategic plan, they often start with a discussion of the content – what the plan should contain. A better starting point, however, is to establish a clear planning process before plunging into the content question. This should be done through the creation of a team that will be responsible for drafting the plan and overseeing the consultation process before the plan is finalized and implemented.

The steps to be taken can be divided into phases: building the leadership team, creating the draft plan, initiating the consultation process, finalizing the plan and carrying it out. In real life, of course, the steps are not so neat and clearly defined; at many points an open and creative process inevitably involves overturning previous decisions and remedying omissions. Some parts of the later stages may overlap with those of the earlier stages. Nevertheless, a map is useful even if the journey contains some unexpected detours or delays. Five stages are described here:

- building the team (structure issues)
- creating the plan (process issues)
- consulting a wider audience
- finalizing the plan
- implementing and reviewing the plan (outcome issues).

Stage 1. Building the team

Finding the leader

Who should lead the process? The leader should be clearly identified and have formal authority, whether she or he is the chief nurse in the health ministry, president of the NNA or the holder of some other nationally recognized position. In general, if the plan is to be adopted as national policy, it may be best to initiate the process within government. The formal position of chief nurse, however, does not always reflect the personal authority of the leader or recognition by others. For example, in a country with a powerful NNA, the most senior nurse in the health ministry may be seen as relatively weak. In some countries, nurses occupy no government positions or only junior ones; these are often the countries with governments that do not understand the need for such plans and are therefore unlikely to initiate or support the process. The initial stimulus for developing the plan may then come from the NNA or other leadership group. Some countries have very decentralized or regionalized systems that do not lend themselves easily to national initiatives. In this case, it may be preferable to develop regional action plans and then bring them together at the national level.

Ultimately, the answer depends on each country's situation, and on finding a leader with the right balance of positional and personal power. No matter who chooses or is given the leadership role, the principle of working through cooperation and consensus helps to minimize fruitless power struggles and constant challenges to the leader's legitimacy.

Supporting the leader

Right from the start, the leader needs access to enough support and funds to establish and maintain a team, and secretarial help to do such tasks as typing letters, booking meeting rooms, arranging travel and so on. The health ministry should be requested to support the project, since the leader cannot be expected to carry it out unaided. If this is impossible, funds may have to be found from other sources inside or outside the country. Group members should be asked to think about this at their first meeting.

Convening the group

The leader should invite interested and influential people to work together on the project. The group may be called a task force, steering group, committee or leadership team. A group of this type may already exist or it may be necessary to start one but, either way, the same process should be followed to ensure that everyone is committed to the project and contributes to it fully.

Sometimes interest can be stimulated by establishing a national committee, chaired by a well known public figure, which then makes recommendations to government; in this case, there must be strong representation of or close liaison with government nurses and other recognized leaders. Alternatively, the NNA, nurses' trade union or other body may set up a group and invite wide participation. In countries with weak nursing leadership, strategic planning sometimes starts with a small, informal group of activists that has no formal authority but can act as a spur to others.

The membership of the group will vary according to national circumstances, but might include some or all of the following:

1. nurses and midwives working in the ministries responsible for health, education and/or labour;
2. officials of other ministries with responsibility for nursing issues;

3. ministry officials with responsibility for planning, human resources and other key functions;
4. representatives of nursing associations and trade unions with nurse members;
5. heads of institutions influential in nursing, such as colleges of nursing, research centres, and WHO collaborating centres;
6. managers of nursing services in hospitals and communities;
7. practitioners of nursing (clinical leaders and innovators);
8. other health professionals, especially doctors;
9. politicians and/or other policy-makers and opinion leaders;
10. citizens' representatives from, for example, community groups, local councils or voluntary organizations; and
11. experts from elsewhere who are working on nursing development in the country, such as advisers from WHO and other intergovernmental and nongovernmental organizations.

The group should be small enough to create a sense of ownership, belonging and trust in its members; the larger the group, the harder this is. The core group should not comprise more than 12 people, who should be committed to attending all meetings; consistency of membership makes the task easier. Not every interest group or influential person can be represented, but ways should be found of involving them all at some stage, such as on subgroups or in the consultation process. The more people that can be involved in this way, the greater the chance of success.

Another issue to resolve is the balance between nurses and nonnurses. Like any group of people with a common understanding and experience, nurses may legitimately discuss their visions, ideals and priorities before sharing them with others. Their conclusions can then be shared and viewed from other perspectives, although nurses should maintain overall leadership of the process.

A further tricky issue is the need to bring together people who may have very different viewpoints. Bringing a variety of perspectives to the group has advantages; it is likely to reflect the diversity of opinion in the wider world and, if well managed, can create stimulating discussion. Nevertheless, tensions may arise from bringing together people with a past history of conflict, especially in countries that have recently undergone rapid political change. A common example is hostility between professional nursing associations and trade unions. The perspectives of both are legitimate and important and both should be considered – not least because anyone who is left out may try to sabotage the project. Excluding one or the other from the group for the sake of a quiet life will ultimately make the task harder, if not impossible. The group should be a genuine attempt to create a consensus, not a vehicle for one faction or another.

Creating the climate

Once the group has been selected and the first meetings are under way, the leader should spend plenty of time helping group members to get to know each other and feel at ease. It is important that they share something of themselves as individuals, not only as representatives or professionals. The leader has a vital role in laying these foundations, and should seek support from trusted colleagues or friends who can help plan the meetings and discuss hopes and fears.

Dealing with the administrative issues

The leader should ask the group to decide what help is needed for the project. She or he should settle at the beginning such practical questions as choosing when and where the meetings will be held; obtaining permission for group members to attend meetings during work time; meeting travel and subsistence expenses; and securing secretarial support, including organizing meetings, taking notes and circulating papers. A budget should be drafted at the beginning, and members should agree on how they will obtain the necessary resources; funding will be needed immediately and later for maintaining the group and publishing, publicizing and debating the plan.

Discussing the need for expert help

The leader and the group may feel they need help with the process, or with particular aspects of the work. Leaders often take on too much by trying to manage both the content of the meetings and the process. They may easily and unwittingly become the scapegoat or lightning conductor for the members' different, sometimes conflicting emotions. It may therefore be valuable to use expert assistance from a facilitator or consultant; this person's role is not to direct the group, but to help it work creatively from a nonpartisan standpoint by managing the process. Such help may be available from WHO or from another organization or person that has no vested interest in influencing the group towards a particular outcome.

Allocating the responsibilities

The leader should ask the group to decide who will be responsible for specific tasks, including chairing the meetings, hosting the meetings, leading subgroups, providing secretarial support, and controlling the budget. For the group to work well, members must understand what is expected of them, and there must be some way of making them accountable for what they do. Formal mechanisms are important, but it is also essential to create a sense of personal ownership and commitment among the members.

Stage 2. Creating the plan

Defining the group's mission

The group needs to reach a shared understanding of its goal, its role and its boundaries before its members can work together effectively. Full and open discussion of the purpose of the project is essential to ensure the members' commitment, understanding and ownership of the task. The leader should start the discussion by outlining the purpose and then inviting comments.

Assessing the situation

One of the group's first tasks is to conduct a brief assessment of the current situation. The resulting map of the environment provides the baseline information on the task that the group is going to tackle. Questions to be considered address the current state of health and health care, the social, political and economic factors likely to influence health in future, the strengths of nursing and the biggest challenges it faces in contributing to health development.

The group needs to identify the sources of the data that it can use to provide a clear and accurate picture. Members' knowledge should be supplemented where possible by any other qualitative and quantitative information available. As well as the country's sources, international organizations such as WHO may have good information. In particular, the Nursing and Midwifery unit in the Regional Office has been working with countries to draw up country nursing and midwifery profiles (see Part I); these make an ideal starting point, as the information summarized in a profile can be reviewed, discussed, and modified or expanded as necessary. The scope of the group's assessment, including the decision on whether to collect new data through surveys or other means, will depend on the resources available to the group, the quality of existing data systems and other factors. The group must strike a balance between the need to be well informed and the need to avoid spending time on gathering data to prove what is already known. The issue of information management can be included in the national action plan.

Describing the vision

WHO and many other organizations have produced statements that describe a vision for nursing – an ideal picture of how it should be. For example, the WHO Director-General *(13)* has provided a view of the role of nurses "not just as active providers of care, meeting the professionally defined needs of passive patients, but as facilitators who help people to take charge of their own health". Other examples have been cited above.

Existing statements are a good starting point for discussion, but group members should also be encouraged to describe their own visions for nursing and its contribution to health. As mentioned, people sometimes have difficulty in getting in touch with their dreams and ideals when they are bogged down in everyday problems, so it is important that the vision both addresses the future and is grounded in the country's social, cultural and political present. It must grow from these roots, rather than be transplanted from elsewhere – otherwise it will be irrelevant and fail to inspire people's commitment, energy, pride and sense of ownership.

Visions are closely tied to people's personal values and beliefs, and some differences are sure to emerge in the group; these should be welcomed and openly explored before the group agrees on the aspects of the visions that overlap or coincide. The group can then formulate its shared vision in a statement that will be embodied in the national action plan and provide the direction and reference point for its goals.

Outlining the options
The vision is likely to be wide ranging. What steps must be taken to realize it? The leader should encourage the group to consider all the possible options for making the vision real, without editing or selecting at this point.

Selecting priorities
The group will have produced many suggestions, but now choices have to be made and priorities recommended. The group must decide what options are the most important. Many actions will need to be taken but it will not be possible to do them all at once. Which should be tackled first? At this stage the group is recommending choices for wider consultation, not making final decisions, but the consultation process will be more productive if some preferred options are set out for discussion.

Analysing the opportunities and difficulties
Setting priorities is one of the most difficult aspects of making an action plan. Depending on their viewpoints or interests, people will have different views about what should be tackled first. Some will argue for the reform of nursing education, while others will advocate the development of clinical practice as the most urgent need. Of course, all such is-

sues must be tackled some time but difficult choices have to be made when resources are limited. Many action plans fail to be implemented because they are unrealistic, containing too many priorities and unachievable goals; people lose faith in such plans.

One useful way to assess how to prioritize the suggested actions is to analyse their chance of success. What are the forces – people, institutions, regulations or finances – that can help or hinder progress on each option? Sometimes an action that everyone favours may be impossible because of circumstances, and sometimes apparently lost causes succeed because support can be mobilized. The group should brainstorm to assess the feasibility of each option, perhaps using a simple planning tool such as force field analysis. Some of this work, as in other stages, can be done by subgroups or in consultation with other people, such as members of different interest groups or other professions.

Agreeing on a draft plan

The possible content of the draft plan is described in more detail below. It could describe the group's vision, the current situation, the proposed priority areas and short-, medium- and long-term goals. Drafting such a plan in committee is difficult; after full discussion by the group, the draft should be prepared by the leader, the secretariat or a small subgroup and then presented to the whole group for comment and final approval.

Stage 3. Consulting a wider audience

Now that the first stage of its work is complete and it has reached consensus on its draft plan, the group can share its ideas with a wider audience. Good communication is crucial at this stage. The group should develop or ask a subgroup or other experts to develop a communication plan that will set out how to publicize the draft, identify the target audience and encourage debate, not only among health professionals but also by the public.

Initially the group may consult a small target group of influential people, such as politicians, the medical association, health care leaders or consumers' associations, to test the water and to win hearts and minds. At the right point, the plan should be disseminated as widely as possible, with the group members explaining and publicizing it. Some countries have done this by sending a printed copy to every qualified nurse, as well as to interest groups. It may be desirable to prepare a simplified version for the non-nursing audience. Nurses may organize public meetings, hold press conferences, and prepare messages for newspapers, magazines and television and radio programmes. Reactions to the plan should be recorded, and written feedback requested by a specific deadline. The consultation process helps:

- to encourage widespread debate on issues that are of great public interest;
- to ensure that all relevant perspectives and views are considered;
- to raise people's awareness and understanding of nursing;
- to attract support from nurses themselves, the public, and politicians and policy-makers;
- to inspire positive thinking and action;
- to highlight areas of difficulty and of special interest;
- to help the leadership group to review, revise and improve the plan; and
- to identify more clearly how the plan can be implemented.

Stage 4. Finalizing the plan

Once the consultation process is complete, the group should meet again to review it and discuss its implications. The group should look at the written responses and any other formal or informal feedback received. It should look again at the plan and review the priorities. Do they still appear feasible in the light of the feedback? At this stage, if the group is confident that the plan will be acceptable to its target audience, it may arrange for the final version to be printed and distributed as widely as possible, as agreed in the communication plan.

The national action plan for nursing needs to contain a detailed work programme. This can be attached to the main document, or issued later as a supplement. It should outline the next steps for the implementation of the short-term priorities, say, for the next year: what is to be done, by whom, when and with what resources. The programme should clearly show how these steps can be linked with or be part of other health care initiatives.

The group may feel that this task belongs to the people who will be responsible for implementing the plan, who may or may not be members of the group itself. If a new group for implementation is more appropriate for the task, it should have overlapping membership with the leadership group and consult it closely. The decision will depend on each country's situation. One option is for the leadership group to become an official (e.g. ministerial) advisory group or steering committee to oversee or advise on implementation. The specific activities in the plan will undoubtedly be the responsibility of many different groups, and these responsibilities need to be set out clearly and negotiated with the groups concerned.

Finally, whether or not the group will continue to meet, its members should celebrate the important journey they have made together.

Stage 5. Implementing the plan

A continuing review process needs to be established for national strategic planning in nursing. No matter how good the plan, it will always need modifying in the light of experience, especially in countries that are undergoing rapid change and where the future is unpredictable. Decisions need to be made – perhaps through recommendations from the planning group – about how and when to assess progress, celebrate the achievements and draw up the next phase of the plan. Evaluating the outcomes of the plan is a difficult but essential issue to tackle.

Implementing the plan is a large and complex topic that cannot fully be explored here. (A further paper is needed, summarizing the extensive experience and literature already available.) It involves great skill in leadership and management, especially the management of change.

What Goes into a National Action Plan?

The content and format of a national action plan for nursing will vary from country to country; there is no perfect blueprint. Depending on the circumstances, a plan could include some or all of the following items:

1. introduction, including messages of support from key figures, such as the health minister, and acknowledgement by name of all the people and organizations that have helped the project;
2. scene setting, including a description of the current situation in health and nursing;
3. a description of the vision for nursing, including its role in various health care settings, and the expected benefits for patients and society;
4. a list of priorities for action, which can be organized in different ways (including grouping under subject headings such as practice, management and education; grouping under functional headings such as PHC and hospital services; or expression as targets, standard statements or goals);
5. the steps to be taken to achieve each priority, including activities, time-scale, resources and responsibility for implementation;

6. a description of the methods to be used to review progress and evaluate outcomes; and
7. contact names and addresses for those who want to become more involved, obtain more information or make comments.

Progress so Far: Some Notes from Countries

Countries are at various stages in the development of national action plans. As mentioned, this is a global movement, not just a European one. Evidence collected by WHO suggests that the scope and purpose of the plans also vary. Some countries, such as the United Kingdom, have developed comprehensive strategies, including targets for practice, education and management. Others take a more narrowly focused starting point; for example, Greece proposes starting with the establishment of a national council for nursing development. In addition, strategies are being developed at subnational or regional level. All four parts of the United Kingdom have developed their own strategies; some cantons in Switzerland have specific nursing plans, as do some provinces of Spain and some *oblasts* in the Russian Federation, such as Tyumen. According to their replies to a 1994 survey conducted by WHO headquarters, the following European countries have developed and adopted plans: the Czech Republic, France, Greece, Hungary, Kazakstan, Latvia, Lithuania, Poland, Sweden, Slovenia, Turkey and the United Kingdom. WHO also knows of development activity in this area in Belarus, Belgium, Croatia, Estonia, Finland, Kyrgyzstan, the Netherlands, Romania, Slovakia and Tajikistan, and work beginning in Armenia, Bulgaria, Georgia, the Republic of Moldova, Turkmenistan, Ukraine and Uzbekistan.

Some examples of the ways in which three countries have tackled the need for strategic planning are given below. The descriptions are not comprehensive or detailed, but intended both to give a flavour of different approaches and to encourage countries to document their own developments in case studies.

England

In 1989, the Nursing Division of the Department of Health (England's equivalent of a health ministry) issued a unique blueprint for the profession entitled *A strategy for nursing (14)*. Designed to be an integral part of government health policy, it was widely circulated and debated within nursing and midwifery. Mindful of the changes facing the professions, a seminar chaired by Anne Poole, then government chief nurse, highlighted ten key issues ranging from the reform of nursing education to the management of standards of practice. A steering group was appointed with wide representation from different branches of the professions. It took the work forward and produced 44 targets for action under the headings of practice, personnel, education, and leadership and management.

After the strategy document was launched there were many changes in NHS policy, producing a host of innovations. The new chief nurse, Yvonne Moores, thought it timely to consider the implications of these changes for nursing and to provide a new framework for nursing, summarized as *A vision for the future: the nursing, midwifery and health visiting contribution to health and health care (15).* This 1993 document set out 5 key areas and 12 targets. The first year's activity was monitored; a survey showed that good progress had been made towards some of the targets, but that more work needed to be done *(16)*. Three project development sites were selected because of their involvement in the implementation of the steering group programme. Each was to examine a different aspect of the national action plan and report on the progress made.

Estonia

Nursing leaders from Estonia were introduced to the idea of national action plans at WHO meetings. They expressed keen interest in working on their own plan and, with encouragement from the chief nurse, Ester Puusepp, the Minister of Social Affairs agreed to include the project in the 1994/1995 medium-term programme of cooperation between WHO and Estonia, thus securing some funds to start the activity. Following discussions, it was agreed that WHO and the chief nurse would arrange a workshop to take forward the ideas and strategies developed at WHO meetings.

Estonia was already developing strong nursing networks. It had established an NNA, and reforms in nursing education and practice were being initiated, sometimes with the help of nurses from neighbouring countries such as Finland and Sweden. These activities were not yet well coordinated, however, and there was no recognized leadership group in nursing. It was decided to use a WHO workshop to create a leadership group. Using the WHO guidelines, the chief nurse identified 20 nursing leaders: nurses, midwives and doctors from health service management, practice, education, the NNA and the Estonia LEMON Group. The group met before the workshop to prepare, and materials were translated into Estonian and circulated in advance. With WHO's help, links had been established with a group of nursing leaders in Finland who were also embarking on the development of a national action plan; these leaders helped to develop the workshop programme and acted as facilitators.

The workshop, held in May 1995 and led by the WHO Regional Adviser for Nursing and Midwifery, Jane Salvage, was evaluated by participants as extremely successful. It helped them to clarify their visions and goals, and to formulate specific objectives. It also introduced them to democratic planning processes and ways of achieving consensus through open discussion and acknowledgement of different perspectives, not only by discussing this in theory but by using it as the working method of the workshop. A group was formally established to carry forward the work, with members drawn from among the participants, and specific themes were identified as priorities for work by subgroups. The participants agreed on a programme of future meetings and decided that the Finnish experts would be consulted on particular issues as the need arose. They forwarded their recommendations to the Minister of Social Affairs, including a request for administrative and financial support in developing the national action plan. They agreed to publicize the outcomes as widely as possible, and both Ms Puusepp and Ms Salvage discussed the issues in the national mass media. (There was widespread interest in nursing at that time as Estonian nurses were threatening strike action over pay.)

The new group met again less than a month later to draw up more detailed plans and establish subgroups to look at education and training, leadership and legislation, terminology in Estonian, and practice standards. A timetable of meetings was agreed until the end of 1995. The chief nurse reported that there had been two radio broadcasts to introduce listeners to the objectives and results of the seminar, which were followed by numerous approving phone calls. Nurses were also invited to give talks in different institutions. The activity looks set to continue and flourish, and has been included in the 1996/1997 medium-term programme of cooperation between WHO and Estonia.

Finland

In 1994, with WHO support, Finnish nurses set up a nursing expert group to develop a strategic plan for their country. It was felt that the achievements and energy of the 1980s, when a strong nursing plan was developed as part of the overall strategy for health for all, were being lost in the 1990s and that a fresh start should be made. The secretariat for the new initiative was based at the National Board for Research and Development in Health (STAKES). Work began with the compilation of a country nursing and midwifery profile for Finland, as suggested by WHO, to bring together systematically data that had not previously been assembled. The completed profile would be disseminated to a wide audience and reviewed at intervals to assess progress. Meetings of the expert group have been held with wide representation – of practice, education, research, administration and regional nurses – to identify and discuss problems.

The strengths of the process were the commitment of those involved, open discussion, good working relationships with the Ministry of Health, and an awareness of possible difficulties. The weaknesses were the already busy lives of the group members, difficulties in collecting data for the profile, an absence of nursing statistics, the interpretation of concepts and the slow (albeit rewarding) process of creating a new culture and building a common vision. The aim was to have a real tool, not a paper exercise, following the guiding principles of patient-centred care, continuity, promotion of health and cost–effectiveness. It was hoped that the draft plan would be completed by the end of 1995. Efforts would then be made to gain acceptance of it through such means as publications and a Delphi survey.

Conclusion

In drawing up a national action plan, it may be useful to look at examples from other countries. Plans drawn up by other health care groups, commercial companies and other organizations may also provide ideas and interesting comparisons, because the steps described here are those that many organizations and groups follow. Articles describing the process of strategic planning can also be helpful; a group may wish to help others by writing about its experiences.

Working on a national action plan for nursing does not solve all the profession's problems, but it helps in many ways. The longest journey starts with a single step, and every traveller should know in which direction to set off – and take a map and compass along.

References

1. *Nursing beyond the year 2000. Report of a WHO Study Group.* Geneva, World Health Organization, 1994 (WHO Technical Report Series, No. 842).
2. *European Conference on Nursing. Report on a WHO meeting.* Copenhagen, WHO Regional Office for Europe, 1989.

3. SALVAGE, J., ED. *Nursing in action. Strengthening nursing and midwifery to support health for all*. Copenhagen, WHO Regional Office for Europe, 1993 (WHO Regional Publications, European Series, No. 48).
4. *Handbook of resolutions and decisions of the World Health Assembly and the Executive Board, Vol. III, 3rd ed. (1985–1992)*. Geneva, World Health Organization, 1993.
5. *Global Advisory Group on Nursing and Midwifery. Report of the second meeting.* Geneva, World Health Organization, 1993 (document WHO/HRH/NUR/93.5).
6. SALVAGE, J. *National action plans for nursing: from vision to implementation*. Copenhagen, WHO Regional Office for Europe, 1993 (document).
7. *First Meeting of Government Chief Nursing Officers and Collaborating Centres on Implications of the HFA Targets for Nursing/Midwifery*. Copenhagen, WHO Regional Office for Europe, 1989 (document EUR/ICP/HSR 334).
8. *Fourth Meeting of European Government Chief Nurses and Collaborating Centres for Nursing and Midwifery. Report on a WHO meeting.* Copenhagen, WHO Regional Office for Europe, 1995 (document EUR/ICP/NURS94 03/MT04).
9. *First WHO Meeting of Government Chief Nurses of the Newly Independent States*. Copenhagen, WHO Regional Office for Europe, 1993 (document ICP/HRH 301(3)).
10. *Second Meeting of Government Chief Nurses of the Newly Independent States*. Copenhagen, WHO Regional Office for Europe, 1994 (document ICP/NURS 94 03/MT02).
11. *Third Meeting of Government Chief Nurses from the Newly Independent States*. Copenhagen, WHO Regional Office for Europe, 1995 (document).
12. *Nursing service policy development manual*. Manila, WHO Regional Office for the Western Pacific, 1994.
13. NAKAJIMA, H. More than ever, we need nurses. *World health*, September–October 1992.
14. *A strategy for nursing. Report of the Steering Committee*. London, Department of Health Nursing Division, 1989.
15. *A vision for the future: the nursing, midwifery and health visiting contribution to health and health care*. Leeds, NHS Management Executive, 1993.
16. *Testing the vision: a report on progress in the first year of "A vision for the future"*. Leeds, NHS Executive, 1995.

5

The role of nurses and midwives in government

Colin Ralph, Jane Salvage & Ruth Ashton

Every country needs nurses and midwives in recognized leadership roles at the national level. Such leadership positions exist or should be created in regulatory bodies, health services, education and research institutions, national professional associations, trade unions, nongovernmental organizations and, by no means least, government. The WHO Regional Office for Europe is often asked to provide guidance on the role and functions of nurses and/or midwives working in government, usually in health ministries or their equivalent. Countries that already have such posts are concerned to make them more effective. Some countries that lack them want help in considering how to establish roles relevant to their particular setting.

WHO policy clearly advocates the strengthening of nursing and midwifery leadership in government at the national level, but to date the Organization has not produced specific guidelines to help countries put the policy into practice. This chapter aims to start filling that gap. It explores the current situation, the existing policy statements, the rationale for such positions, their functions and some of the issues that arise. The first part of the chapter looks more specifically at the government chief nurse, while the second part focuses on the contribution of midwifery to policy-making and action at the national level – a linked but separate debate. Chief nurses may carry the responsibility for midwifery in some countries, while others have chief midwife positions. Nursing and midwifery are separate professions in some countries and united in others, and the issues raised in the two parts of this chapter are largely relevant to both. We take no view on the desirability of having a chief midwife or similar position, but the principles advocated will be of help in any debate on the nature of that function, once its importance has been recognized. Such debate should take place in every country. For the purpose of this chapter, however, the specific issues relating to midwifery must not detract from the importance of the debate on the government chief nurse.

Another question that flows logically from these debates is the issue of central government and its role in increasingly decentralized health care systems. Should WHO be advocating the need for nursing and midwifery positions in government at a time when many ministries are being reduced in size and scope, and are changing their roles in dramatic ways? We address this question below.

The Current Situation

The term chief nurse is used here as a generic title to denote the most senior nurse in government – in other words, a person employed in a nursing capacity in the health ministry (or equivalent) and providing a focal point for nursing (and possibly midwifery) within the ministry (see pp. 25–29 in Part I). Some health ministries also, or as an alternative, employ nurses and/or midwives in certain departments to work on specific programmes or to provide advice and direction on specific issues. Most often they are found in ministry departments of education, human resources, health services or maternal and child health. These nurses and midwives – important though their positions are – are not the focus of this chapter, which is concerned primarily with the issue of professional leadership.

The title role and functions of the government chief nurse vary between countries. They are influenced by many factors, including the country's political agenda, the attitude of permanent officials of the ministry such as the chief medical officer, the strength of organized nursing and midwifery and the regard in which they are held. Another major influence is the country's administrative structure, which affects the strength or weakness of central government functions. Such factors have been responsible, in whole or in part, for the huge diversity between countries. At best, some ministry nursing and midwifery positions have great authority and responsibility; at worst, there are no such positions and nursing and midwifery have no formal means of contributing to the work of government.

It is difficult to give accurate information here about the current position in the European Region. Some countries have stable chief nurse posts, but in many others – especially at this time of rapid political and social change – posts are being disestablished, re-established soon after, or left vacant, or their functions temporarily handled through ad hoc arrangements. According to data available at the time of writing, the Member States of the WHO European Region can be divided into several broad groups, although the categories are loosely defined and sometimes overlap:

- thirteen countries with ministries that have maintained as a tradition or recently reintroduced a chief nurse post with a recognized executive function (Croatia, the Czech Republic, Denmark, Hungary, Iceland, Israel, Poland, Slovakia, Slovenia, Spain, Sweden, Turkey and the United Kingdom);
- four countries with a chief nurse in the ministry whose role is mainly advisory (Belgium, Finland, Malta and the Netherlands);
- eight countries whose ministry's structure was based on the Soviet model, in which the post of chief specialist for nursing was common (and often occupied by a feldsher), and that have retained or reintroduced this role (Estonia, Georgia, Kyrgyzstan, Latvia, Lithuania, Tajikistan, Turkmenistan and Uzbekistan);
- eight countries whose ministries have no chief nurse post or unit but have one or more nurses or midwives working in other departments (Albania, Bulgaria, France, Ireland, Italy, Norway, Portugal and Romania);
- two countries with federal systems, authority decentralized to provinces or cantons, and only small ministries with no nursing post (Germany and Switzerland); and
- thirteen countries with no nurses or midwives employed in the health ministry at all (Armenia, Austria, Azerbaijan, Belarus, Bosnia and Herzegovina, Greece, Kazakstan, Luxembourg, the Republic of Moldova, the Russian Federation, San Marino, The Former Yugoslav Republic of Macedonia and Ukraine).

It is interesting to compare these WHO data with those collected in the global study of chief nurse positions in national ministries of health by Splane & Splane *(1)*. Between 1985 and 1993, they noted the existence of these positions in health ministries in 19 countries in Europe and another 79 worldwide. At first sight, the number may seem to have recently declined in Europe. Splane & Splane, however, apply their "chief nursing officer" (CNO) broadly, to nurses carrying positions with a variety of designations and with considerable differences in reporting relationships and responsibilities.

Splane & Splane *(1)* sum up well the difficulty of mapping any trends in the creation or dissolution of chief nurse posts:

> If the list [of countries with a CNO] were of all countries that had established a CNO position at any time in their history, it would have been considerably longer. ... This is an indication of the non-static nature of the CNO Movement: at a given time CNO positions are in the process of being established; a number of existing CNO positions are performing near the optimum level; and some are threatened with downgrading or elimination.

In the European Region, two possible trends can be discerned, and we offer them here as tentative conclusions that require much more extensive analysis. First, in some western countries, the introduction of general management structures and the increasing predominance of career administrators have weakened health professionals' leadership in ministries. Conversely, in some of the CCEE and NIS, the role of chief nurse is gaining new strength in response to the perceived urgent need to improve the quality of health care.

Many health ministries, as mentioned above, employ nurses and/or midwives in different departments or divisions; indeed, some are employed by other ministries such as those responsible for labour or education. Important as these roles may be, they are not the main subject of this chapter. People in these positions are rarely, if ever, in charge of their own department and very often report to a doctor; they do not take the lead in nursing/midwifery policy or management, but contribute to other functions or programmes. Splane & Splane *(1)*, calling this arrangement the dispersal model, summarize the situation well:

> [These nurses] may exercise some influence on policy and management as part of multidisciplinary teams and, in certain situations, they may be the team or programme leader. Although relatively senior in such instances, they remain at a distance from central decision-making. Moreover, with the nurses dispersed throughout its various programme units, the ministry lacks a focal point for nursing.

In some countries, those in such positions have tried to strengthen the voice of nursing through a network of all nursing or midwifery colleagues in ministries. This seldom seems to succeed, for various reasons:

- such a network is difficult to organize and maintain;
- it is not encouraged by other colleagues, who see it as divisive;
- there is no clear authority or leadership, and anyone attempting to take the lead may be viewed with suspicion; and
- people's loyalty lies primarily with their own team or division.

The post of chief midwife is found in a few countries, but more often the person with responsibility for midwifery reports to the chief nurse, or is based in a ministry department of maternal and child health reporting to a chief obstetrician. According to replies to a 1994 survey by WHO headquarters, only two countries in the Region reported having a chief midwife post (Armenia and the United Kingdom), and one reported having a combined chief nurse/chief midwife post (the Czech Republic). The subject requires further research.

Existing Policy Statements

The linked issues of professionals' leadership positions in government and the nursing and midwifery contribution to developing health plans and policy have received some attention from WHO and other agencies in recent years. In 1989 the World Health Assembly urged WHO Member States to encourage and support the appointment of nursing personnel in senior leadership and management positions, and to facilitate their participation in planning and implementing the country's health activities *(2)*. Three years later, the Health Assembly adopted resolution WHA45.5 *(2)* urging Member States "to strengthen managerial and leadership capabilities and reinforce the positions of nursing and midwifery personnel in all health care settings and at all levels of service, including the central and local services of health ministries ...", and "to ensure that the contribution of nursing and midwifery is reflected in health policies".

These issues were already being explored worldwide, as well as in the European Region. The first WHO European Conference on Nursing, held in Vienna in 1988, recognized the need for nurses to develop roles as partners in decision-making on the planning and management of national health services *(3)*. Subsequent international meetings of the European anglophone and russophone networks of government chief nurses, which WHO founded in 1989 and 1993, respectively, debated this at length and produced further statements. (The networks are now known as LINK.) In addition, the Fourth Meeting of European Government Chief Nurses and WHO Collaborating Centres for Nursing and Midwifery, which was held in 1994 with participants from 32 Member States (see Annex 3), urged countries to ensure that the professional and corporate contribution of nursing leaders was recognized and encouraged in ministries of health *(4)*.

Nursing leaders from the CCEE and NIS, where nursing is in general less autonomous and less respected than in other countries of the

Region, are now paying particular attention to the issue. The person responsible for nursing in health ministries is often a doctor, and it is not yet seen as axiomatic that nurses and midwives should take the lead in policy- and decision-making for their profession, although this is gradually changing. The First WHO Meeting of Government Chief Nurses of the Newly Independent States, held in Kazakstan in 1993, identified the need for the position of chief nurse in ministries of health and for each country to develop a national action plan for nursing (see Annex 1). The Second Meeting, held in 1994, recommended that each country establish or, where appropriate, enlarge the nursing department of each health ministry *(5)*. The Third Meeting, held in 1995, was the first attended by teams of leaders from all 15 NIS, and again the issue was prominent. The meeting statement (see Annex 4) said that the development of nursing and midwifery required strong leadership from within. Chief nurse and chief midwife positions in the health ministry must be occupied by a qualified nurse, midwife or feldsher and have appropriate staffing and budgets. Where no such positions exist, they should be created as soon as possible.

Other leading international organizations have made similar recommendations. For example, in 1991 ICN urged governments to recognize and capitalize on the experience of nursing managers, and to educate nurses to fill management roles at the country level *(6)*. In 1993 the Commonwealth Secretariat *(7)*, in its action plan for nursing, identified the need to recognize and strengthen the government-level nursing policy function in each country, in order to "provide informed intelligence on nursing practice and management to ministers and others". It stated:

> Nurses and midwives must play a full part in key policy and planning decisions. The knowledge which comes from their practice places them in a privileged position to bring to decision-making at ministerial and senior government level, and to boards of management of health services in the public and private sectors, that perspective of service delivery without which decisions are often flawed.

This followed recommendations made by the Commonwealth chief nurses and professional associations at their 1992 conference in Malta.

Since the issue has so frequently been debated, and been the subject of recommendations and statements, the question arises as to the impact of all this discussion on actual practice. This is difficult, perhaps impossible, to summarize. In the last few years, chief nurse posts have been re-established or strengthened in at least eight European countries, and perhaps part of the credit for that can be given to WHO for its continuing advocacy. Such a claim is anecdotal, however; almost no research has been carried out on the role or the trends in its development. A notable exception is the study by Splane & Splane mentioned above *(1)*. They collected data using a variety of methods over an eight-year period, including visits to 50 countries and interviews with over 90 past and current chief nurses. They concluded that all governments should establish a senior nursing position in their ministries of health, as the requisite means of promoting the best utilization of nurses in improving the nation's health.

Splane & Splane also traced the history of the role. They note the influence of WHO in what they call the "CNO Movement", and how nursing's position in WHO itself has waxed and waned at different times *(1)*:

> WHO continues to represent both the greatest challenge and the greatest opportunity for advances in nursing and for the forward advance of the CNO Movement. … The goal is to restore WHO's recognition of the role of nursing in world health to the place it held in WHO's first quarter century.

The Chief Nurse

Rationale for the role

WHO and other organizations clearly advocate the need for chief nurse positions in government. It would be inappropriate, however, to propose a blueprint for the role and functions that could be applied in each country. A prescriptive approach could reduce the potential success of such roles, as national, political and cultural considerations must be taken into account. Nevertheless, we set out here the rationale for the creation and continuing existence of chief nurses, with a description of the key elements that endow them with the necessary characteristics to influence health policy and lead and develop the profession. At this stage of the debate, generalities are needed, to capture the important elements that justify the need for the role. More specific questions (such as whether the chief nurse should have executive responsibility or an advisory role) are secondary. The primary issue is securing an effective nursing contribution to health policy and the development of nursing, and therefore to the people's health.

There can be only one rational argument for the existence of a government chief nurse: that the nursing profession makes a major contribution to people's health and health care and is therefore an integral and vital asset to the health care system. It follows that health ministries should recognize this asset and secure the contribution of suitably experienced and able nurses at a senior level to translate the nursing contribution to health into policy terms. This will ensure that a nursing contribution enriches the development and implementation of health policy, and the management of health systems.

The nature of the nursing contribution to health care varies between health systems but, in every country, disease and ill health are widespread, health promotion is necessary to improve health gain, and people of all ages who are ill and/or vulnerable require skilled nursing care in addition to medical attention. Various factors determine the contribution that the nursing and midwifery profession is permitted to make in each country; these include the traditional role of the profession, its relationship with the medical profession and its degree of public recognition. In turn, these matters are influenced by the position of women in society and their access to educational opportunity and to senior positions in the health, social and political systems, as well as the degree to which the profession has been able to organize itself as a collective body with agreed aims and plans. While the nursing profession may have a different history in each country, the restraining factors are common to all countries. The constant need for nursing requires health policy to be sensitive to people's needs for such care, and provides the rationale for establishing a chief nurse post in every health ministry.

The rationale requires further elaboration to clarify the purpose of the role. This is to ensure a nursing contribution to the development of health policy, to lead the profession, and to assist the ministry in its work for the benefit of people who depend on nursing when their health is compromised. The purpose is not to advance or represent the profession at the ministry for the sake of the profession. A chief nurse is likely to have an effect in advancing the profession as a leader of nursing in her or his country, but this is secondary, and justified only if it serves the primary purpose of the role. Various secondary effects of a chief nurse's work may benefit the health system and the profession, such as systematic information gathering through networks, testing the ministry's proposed plans with other leaders of the profession, and improving education or working conditions for nurses. Nevertheless, the primary purpose of the role must always be clear. Any proposed initiative by a chief nurse should be tested by asking whether it is in the public interest, to benefit society. Put more clearly, the primary purpose is to serve the public good, not the interests of the profession.

Other arguments may be used to justify the role of chief nurse, such as the large number of nurses in a country, the cost of nursing as a proportion of the health budget, and the need for nursing to have a voice at the health ministry. These arguments alone provide no real justification for the role. The nature of the nursing contribution to the health care system provides the single rational argument, the only one likely to be sustained in the face of political, administrative or other challenges.

The ministry of health

The ministry of health is a complex environment in which the chief nurse must learn to function effectively. In many cases she or he has had no previous experience of government service, having often been appointed from a senior health service or education post. In countries where the role is not yet established, very few, if any, potential chief nurses have experience of work in government. This creates a special need to prepare nurses for the role, and to support and develop chief nurses once in post. The following factors are some of those that influence their work.

In some countries, politicians appoint senior officials; thus, as politicians change, officials may also change. The political agenda largely determines the priorities and plans of the health ministry. Permanent officials strongly influence how and by whom the work of the ministry is carried out, how officials are appointed and how the work of departments is supported. Other professional staff – such as the chief medical officer or the head of human resources – also influence the work and priorities of the ministry and its staff. Ministry employees are appointed to serve the government, and are required to be loyal to the government and, often, to promote its policies. In addition, government servants are expected to adopt the values of government service. This can create a particular challenge for chief nurses, who need to interpret professional events and dilemmas in the world outside the ministry to the people within it. A chief nurse who is perceived within the ministry as an advocate of the profession – and not the public good – may see her or his contribution disregarded or role endangered.

These circumstances contribute to a challenging environment and a complex set of working relationships. They can also create conflict for the chief nurse. For example, how does she or he respond when the ambitions of the government do not coincide with those of the profession? This illustrates the complexity of the role and the personal tensions it can generate. The chief nurse is a government servant, but also needs to be perceived as a leader by the nursing community in order to influence professional development. Reconciling these different and sometimes apparently conflicting perspectives and expectations requires great personal skill.

The positional power of the chief nurse within the structure and organization of the health ministry is of considerable importance. A chief nurse appointed to a senior level, with access to the most senior officials and, critically, to the minister, is more effective than one appointed to a lower level with no such access. The relative influence of the division or department in which the chief nurse is based is another factor. Often linked with this, the size of the budget and the extent of administrative and professional staff support are also important influences on effectiveness.

A factor of increasing importance is the changing role of ministries of health. Sociopolitical trends such as the decline of communism and the dominance of right-wing economic ideology have combined – rightly or wrongly – to discredit the role of the state and central government in civic life. All over Europe, the power to make policy, hold the purse strings and manage health services is being devolved to lower, more local levels. Even where ministries have retained nominal control, this may simply be disregarded, especially in the current volatile state of some countries, which have weak or even bankrupt ministries that lack the means to enforce their decisions. Nearly all ministries have made heavy staff cuts in recent years, and nursing and midwifery positions have been among the casualties in some countries. The ministry's and the chief nurse's authority to establish policy and insist that specific measures are carried out nationwide may well be seen as anachronistic and undesirable, and may be challenged. Increasingly, concerted action is achieved not by decree but by negotiation, consensus and alliance building. Ironically, it is also true that coordination and inspiration from the centre, and even control in specific areas where public safety and welfare are involved (such as educational and practice standards, or the registration of practitioners) are even more needed today.

The issues are too complex to be discussed at length here, but the implications for nursing leadership roles should be noted and debated further. In particular, how can the right balance be struck between desirable local autonomy and fragmentation or anarchy, and between national visions, goals and frameworks and the best local solutions? A balance also needs to be struck between achieving the goals of the government of the day, and achieving those agreed by consensus among all stake-holders. Ideally, the chief nurse works not as the top of a hierarchy but as a coordinator, facilitator and catalyst of the country's nursing leaders.

Role and functions of the chief nurse

Some of the influences on the chief nurse's role have already been discussed. In some countries, the chief nurse has nursing colleagues to provide assistance, and other staff to manage. In others, she or he may have executive responsibilities in addition to those for nursing, or an executive nursing role rather than an advisory one. Splane & Splane *(1)* give a full description of these two models: the executive and the advisory. It would not be appropriate to select one as a WHO recommendation, since neither would suit all countries. The following description of the chief nurse's role and functions is based on the primary purpose described earlier, and should be seen as a check-list to be reviewed, applied and adjusted according to the needs of each country.

The reader should note one further point before studying the check-list. The creation or existence of chief nurse posts do not guarantee their continuation. Even in countries where the role is well established, the need for its existence is challenged from time to time and there is no room for complacency. Strategies are required not only to enable posts to be created, but also to secure their continuing existence and effectiveness. The development of such strategies is not directly the subject of this chapter, but it is a matter that requires attention, and one key element must be emphasized here. The chief nurse should recognize that her or his contribution must be seen to be of value to ministers, officials and the work of the ministry. She or he will encounter a number of key people inside the ministry, as well as others outside, who have differing expectations. Along with the environment and relationships within the ministry itself, this poses a particular challenge: one way to meet it is to create alliances within and outside the ministry that will enable her or him to operate effectively, to meet these conflicting expectations, and to sustain the role in the face of any threat.

The check-list below sets out the key functions and the most desirable arrangements for the chief nurse to make a positive impact on the health ministry and its work. It may take time for each element to be achieved, and stages may need to be identified to improve and strengthen the role over time. Patience and determination are just two of the qualities required for sustained success. The check-list is not exhaustive and is presented for debate and refinement. It may be used as a basis for drawing up a post description.

Check-list

The chief nurse is the leading nursing expert in the health ministry and is responsible for providing the professional nursing contribution to health policy, planning and programmes. The chief nurse leads the development of the profession in the interests of health care, and assists the ministry in developing and managing the health care system. As a minimum, the role has advisory and consultative, leadership, intelligence-gathering and liaison functions. Further, specific organizational requirements are necessary if the chief nurse is to make an effective contribution.

The advisory and consultative function
The chief nurse advises and is consulted by:

1. the health minister and senior officials on all matters relating to nursing;
2. the health minister and senior officials on all aspects of proposed health policy, plans and programmes that have implications for nursing; and
3. ministers and officials of other ministries (such as those for welfare, education and the environment) on all issues that may relate to or have implications for nursing.

The leadership function – strategy
The chief nurse provides:

1. leadership in the development of strategies and of a national action plan for nursing to increase the positive impact of nursing on health, acting as convenor of the national group of nursing leaders;
2. an expert nursing contribution to national health policy, plans and programmes; and
3. strategic leadership and overall direction for the profession through alliances and influence.

The leadership function – practice
The chief nurse leads:

1. the preparation of a statement of purpose for nursing to promote the optimal contribution of nurses to the health system;
2. initiatives to establish criteria for assessing, improving and researching standards of nursing practice and care; and
3. initiatives to establish the effect of nursing on health gain and the effectiveness of nursing practice and care.

The leadership function – education
The chief nurse leads:

1. initiatives to ensure that the standard of nursing education is at least comparable to that of education for other health professions, and that it meets WHO recommendations and other appropriate international directives and guidelines;

2. initiatives to ensure the necessary focus on primary and secondary health care; and
3. initiatives to improve standards of schools and colleges of nursing and the preparation of teachers of nursing.

The leadership function – legislation, regulation and registration
The chief nurse leads:

1. initiatives to ensure that new laws relating to nursing are prepared and existing laws reformed, to enable the potential nursing contribution to health care to be realized in full;
2. initiatives to collaborate with the medical profession and others to ensure that nurses' scope of practice enhances and develops, not constrains, the nursing role;
3. initiatives to assist the profession's regulatory body in developing a code of conduct and practice and, where a regulatory body does not exist, to promote its creation; and
4. initiatives to ensure that a register is maintained of all nurses trained in the country and all nurses migrating from other countries, and that it is kept up to date and developed as a tool for human resource planning.

The intelligence-gathering function
The chief nurse:

1. receives and interprets information from within the health ministry, and from other ministries when relevant, on proposed health policy, plans and programmes;
2. receives and interprets statistical and other information on health services and human resources in health care, including medical, nursing and auxiliary staff;
3. receives and interprets information from the profession, the health and educational systems and other sources relevant to the range of the chief nurse's functions; and
4. alerts the minister and officials to events within or beyond the profession that may require attention, including relevant policies and recommendations produced by national and international organizations.

The liaison function
The chief nurse liaises with:

1. the health minister and officials to ensure an adequate flow of information;
2. other ministries as necessary;

3. leaders of the profession's representative, educational and regulatory organizations;
4. key nursing and other staff throughout the health system to ensure an adequate flow of information; and
5. international organizations relating to nursing, including WHO and ICN, and chief nurses in health ministries in other countries.

Organizational requirements

To work effectively, the chief nurse has requirements of an organizational kind. These include authority, access, organizational position and support as set out below.

Authority

The chief nurse should have – and be seen by others within the ministry to have – the authority and approval of the minister and/or the most senior officials to carry out the full range of functions of the role.

Access

The chief nurse requires access to:

1. the minister and senior officials, including the chief medical officer on all professional matters and on matters that may have implications for nursing;
2. all papers and other sources of information, both within the ministry and elsewhere, relating to the chief nurse's range of functions;
3. staff of the ministry of health and other ministries whose work is related to the range of functions;
4. leaders and organizations outside the ministry as necessary;
5. nurses and others within the health system as necessary; and
6. all papers and other sources of information from international and other national organizations relating to nursing.

Organizational position

The chief nurse should:

1. report to the most senior permanent official within the ministry;
2. be a member of the most senior group within the ministry that is responsible for determining health policy and making decisions regarding the health system;
3. be a member of the group responsible for managing the health services; and
4. be a member of all groups that consider policy issues relating to the chief nurse's range of functions and that deal with international and national matters that may have implications for nursing.

Support
The chief nurse requires the following kinds of support:

1. assistance with role and functions from other nurses;
2. assistance from computer and information technology, statistical and other experts, and administrative, library, secretarial and clerical staff; and
3. adequate financing to meet the requirements of the role and range of functions, and the power to authorize expenditure from the budget.

Personal characteristics
It is inappropriate to be too prescriptive about the characteristics of chief nurses. Effectiveness is often a personal matter, and success in a role depends not only on formal qualifications and preparation but also on the person's intuitive, intellectual, interpersonal and presentation skills. The following is therefore simply a guide to the desirable background and characteristics of potential chief nurses:

1. education in nursing-related studies to at least degree level;
2. experience in clinical nursing in primary and secondary health care;
3. responsibility, including experience in managerial and/or educational posts responsible for nursing services;
4. interest in nursing practice, education, management and research, and in health policy;
5. intellectual ability to conceptualize and analyse options and issues;
6, political understanding of systems and processes and the politics of organizations;
7. intuitive skill – a developed sense of intuition and sensitivity to both hidden and disclosed agendas;
8. interpersonal understanding and the ability to develop collaborative relationships, secure consensus and develop alliances;
9. facilitation skills – the ability to lead a team towards shared goals and to help the team solve problems;
10. communication – the ability to communicate oral and written messages in a succinct and persuasive manner; and
11. presentation skills – the ability to speak with authority and to represent the profession with impact and influence.

The position of chief nurse is of great importance to ministries, health systems and the profession. Meeting the demands of the role requires the support of key people within the health ministry, and sufficient authority and assistance. A chief nurse cannot succeed alone; the support, assistance and cooperation of others are needed. The role of chief nurse; her or his relationships with others in the ministry, the profession and beyond; the culture of ministries of health; and the effect of often conflicting priorities and demands call for exceptional ability. The contribution of chief nurses is critical to the development and advancement of the profession for the good of people in every country. It is hoped that this chapter will assist in further refining the rationale for and the key elements of this important role and its functions.

Contribution of Midwifery to Policy-making and Action at National Level

This second section of the chapter explores and clarifies the contribution of midwifery to policy-making and action relating to maternity services at the national level in health ministries or their equivalents. It sets out the arguments for and elements of the role of an identifiable midwifery function at that level, to facilitate the fulfilment of national goals for safe motherhood and perinatal care.

Midwifery should be a particular and recognizable service within the maternity services, and it should be available to all women: this is the primary principle. No argument is made here for or against having a chief midwife at the ministerial or policy-making level. A decision about the nature of the person or people who provide a midwifery focus to ministers or policy-makers depends on a number of different factors, many of which are contained in the analysis of the rationale for and the role and functions of the chief nurse. Nothing in this section should be seen to detract from the contribution that other health professionals, such as nurses or doctors, could or should make to the development of national priorities, policies or plans for the provision of maternity care.

Background

WHO global and regional policies for health, including that of women and children, contain a strong commitment to safe motherhood and perinatal care, and stress their priority in global, regional and national health care programmes. The WHO policy for health for all, and the safe motherhood initiative and global and regional policies associated with it, explicitly acknowledge the role of the midwife in achieving these priorities.

The 1989 World Health Assembly urged that nursing and midwifery be strengthened to support the strategy for health for all in resolution WHA42.27 *(2)*. The 1992 Health Assembly built on this foundation in resolution WHA45.5 *(8)*, which restated its commitment to the promotion of nursing and midwifery as essential health services in all countries for the development and improvement of all health for all strategies. The development of a strategy that recognizes and promotes midwifery as an essential part of the maternity care would be a major component of a national strategy for providing effective maternity services. The Assembly identified key activities and called for action plans to incorporate them.

The new WHO *Mother–baby package (9)* is a practical guide to the operational and clinical processes that jointly lead to the improvement of pregnancy outcomes. It sees midwifery skills as a vital component of these processes. The document shows that implementation of the processes requires the development of a national policy framework and action plan, and that the plan's success depends on high-level national commitment, including that of political leaders and policy-makers at the highest levels. These principles are important in the provision of maternity services in any country, irrespective of the current state of its services and outcomes, or its socioeconomic position.

The safe and healthy outcome of every pregnancy should be a major priority in the health care policy of every country. The *Mother–baby package* identifies the task that countries face if this objective is to be achieved *(9)*:

> The challenge which now confronts decision-makers, health care planners and managers, and health care providers is to ensure that every pregnant woman has access to high quality essential care. ... In order to ensure that as many pregnant women as possible have access to the essentials of care, a balance will have to be achieved between what is absolutely critical for all women and what would be ideal if circumstances permitted.

Every country is responsible for providing universally accessible, high-quality maternity care to each childbearing woman. As part of this responsibility, each country needs to define its priorities and rationalize the service accordingly. The provision of care to an individual woman is brought about through a complex mixture of policy, management, operational and clinical processes, and of the skills of many different people, both in and outside the health care system, including policy-makers and planners, managers, health professionals, educators, support workers and others. The effectiveness of the service depends on achieving cohesion between all these different elements. The ultimate responsibility for ensuring this cohesion rests with political leaders and policy-makers.

Government staff or policy-makers would benefit in several important ways from an identifiable midwifery contribution when priorities, policies and plans for maternity care are being addressed.

Role of midwifery

Midwifery is an integral part of a maternity service that is capable of achieving national goals for maternal and perinatal care. It is an essential health service for the support and development of strategies for the safety of mothers and the health of the nation. People with midwifery skills are involved across the full spectrum of maternity care, from primary to tertiary level, which provides a unique overview of service provision. The skills of each midwifery practitioner play a key role in the achievement of overall national objectives for maternity services, and in the processes involved in achieving satisfactory outcomes to individual pregnancies.

Contribution to the development of policies, priorities and plans

In any country the provision and shape of maternity services are defined and determined at the national or policy-making level. As an essential component of the maternity services, the provision and shape of the midwifery service should also be defined and determined at this level and must reflect the needs of the maternity service. Success will be impossible without a discrete, identifiable midwifery contribution to all aspects of the development of a national strategy and plan of action for maternity care.

Midwifery should play a significant role in defining priorities for the maternity service. It is well placed to assist in defining priorities against the resources available, and in rationalizing the provision of care to achieve optimum results.

Midwives' involvement in the full spectrum of maternity care places them in direct contact with all personnel in the service and all the operational processes that support it. Midwives provide a unique knowledge of the strengths and weaknesses of the service. If policy-makers are to build into their strategies the processes to achieve cohesion, they will need to utilize midwives' experience interpreted through a national-level midwifery function.

Midwifery provides an understanding of factors that affect the outcomes of differing levels and types of care and has a role in interpreting the significance of maternity care data. Midwifery can assist in defining the differing but complementary roles of other health professionals, including doctors, and can contribute to discussions of national staffing and skill needs and decisions.

Contribution to plans for maternity services

Fig. 1 provides a framework for the systematic development of the issues that will shape the type of strategy and plans to meet each coun-

Fig. 1. Framework for developing a national policy, priorities and an action plan for maternity services

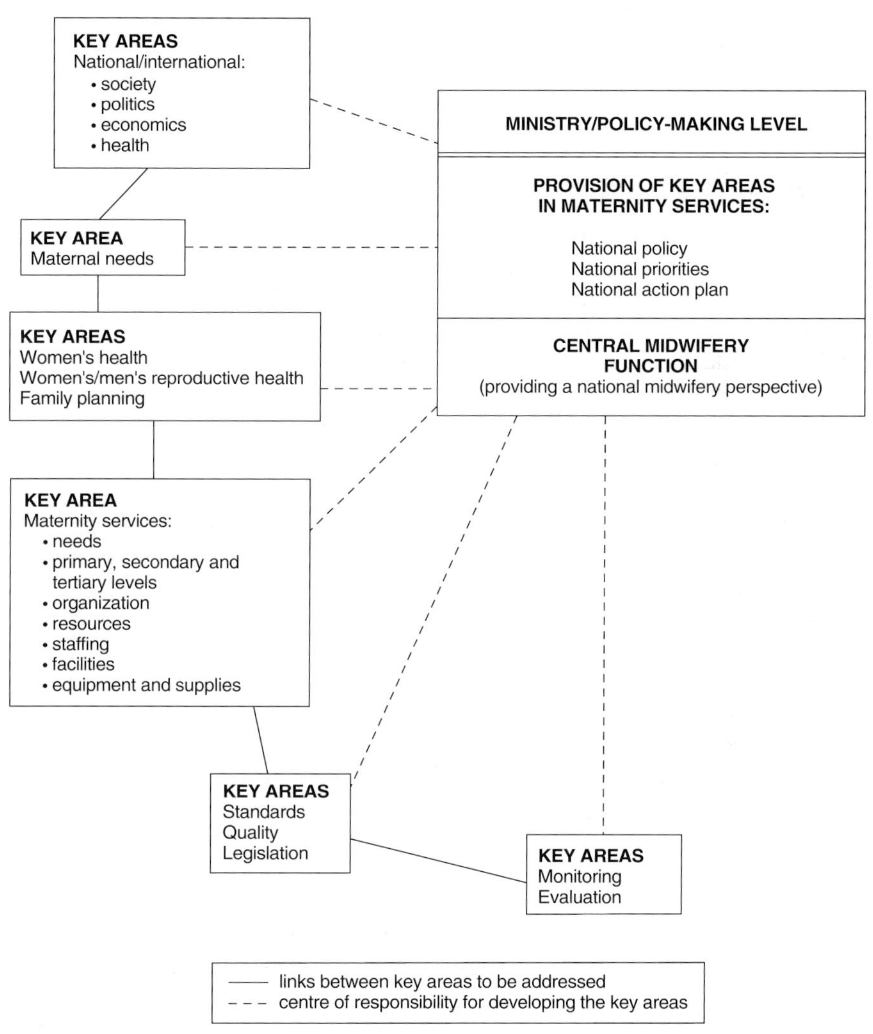

try's needs for maternity services. It gives key areas to be addressed at the national level in the development of policies, priorities and plans and the process for implementing them. The following list from the *Mother–baby package (9)* indicates some activities that should form a part of this work (Table 1):

1. definition of national policy and guidelines
2. analysis of the situation and assessment of needs
3. preparation of national action plans
4. estimation of costs of implementation
5. identification of sources of support
6. preparation of detailed implementation plans
7. implementation of interventions
8. monitoring and evaluation.

Table 1. Key areas and activities for a midwifery contribution at the national level

Key areas	Activities
Maternal needs	Situation analysis and needs assessment
Women's health	
Women's and men's reproductive health	
Family planning	
Maternity services	
Standards and quality	
Monitoring and evaluation	
Provision of maternity services: national policy, priorities and action plan	Definition of national policy and policy, priorities and action plan guidelines Estimation of costs of implementation Preparation of detailed implementation plans Implementation of interventions Monitoring and evaluation

Contribution to a midwifery action plan

The concept and process of developing national action plans for nursing and midwifery are described more fully in Chapter 4. The action plan for midwifery will be an effective component of the national action plan for maternity services if:

- it is developed at or supported by the national level;

- it reflects national policies, priorities and plans for the provision of a maternity service aimed at improving maternal and perinatal outcomes; and
- it strengthens midwifery in support of safe or safer childbirth.

Clearly, the responsibility for the national midwifery action plan lies at ministerial or policy-making level. The development of the plan requires a comprehensive knowledge and understanding of midwifery and the midwifery service, and the part each plays in the provision of services. This knowledge should be available through an identifiable midwifery function at the national level. The implementation of the plan depends on the extent to which it is realistic and accurately reflects the service and circumstances of people with midwifery skills. The midwifery contribution to planning has an important part to play in achieving such realism.

Resolution WHA45.5 *(8)* calls on Member States to take eight steps in strengthening nursing and midwifery in support of strategies for health for all. These steps can easily be recast as activities for developing midwifery:

1. identifying needs for midwifery services, followed by the assessment of the role and utilization of midwives;
2. strengthening managerial and leadership capabilities and reinforcing the position of midwifery personnel at all levels of service, including the central and local services of health ministries and the local authorities responsible for the programmes concerned;
3. enacting legislation where necessary or taking other appropriate measures to ensure good midwifery services;
4. strengthening education in midwifery, adapting educational programmes to the strategy and revising them where appropriate in order to meet the changing care needs of the population;
5. promoting and supporting health services research that will ensure the optimal contribution of midwifery to health care delivery;
6. ensuring appropriate working conditions to sustain the motivation of personnel and improve the quality of services;
7. ensuring the allocation of adequate resources (financial, human and logistic) for midwifery activities; and
8. ensuring that the contribution of midwifery is reflected in policies on maternity services.

Fig. 2 shows a framework for the development of a national action plan for midwifery based on these activities. It provides for a systematic and comprehensive approach to key areas that should be developed within

Fig. 2. Framework for developing a national action plan for midwifery

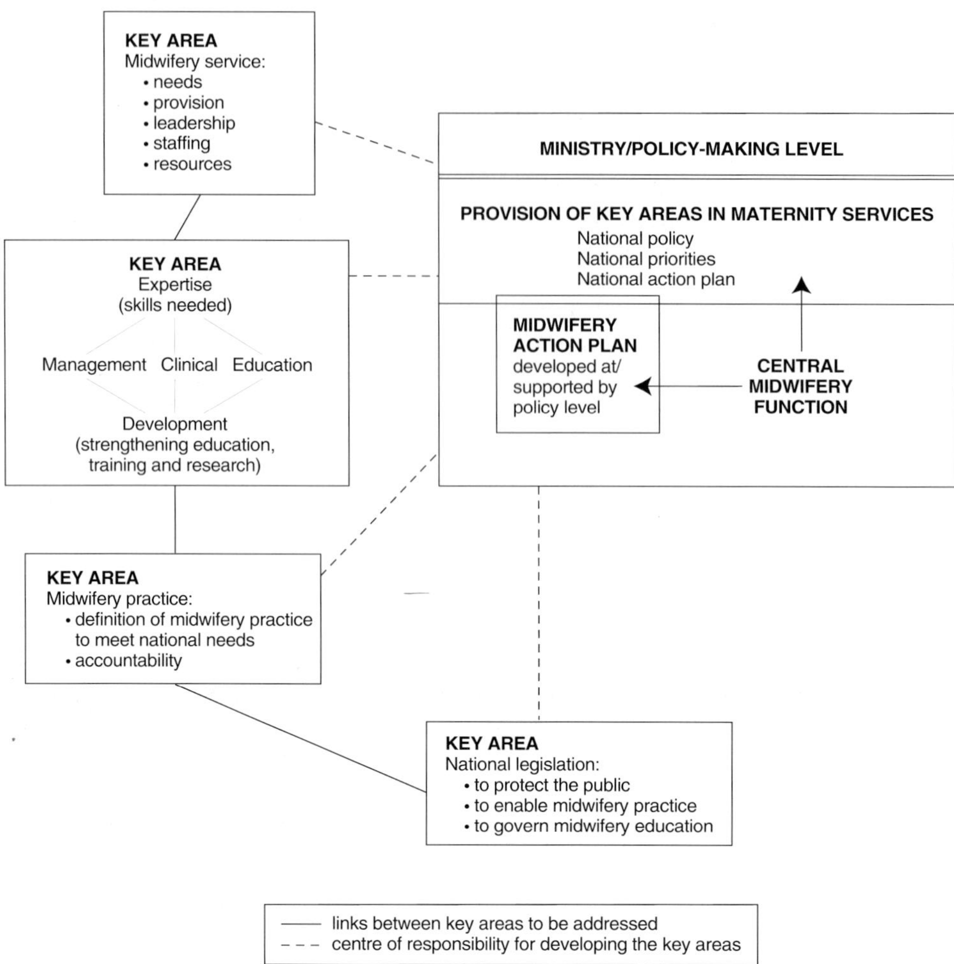

the plan if the provision of maternity care is to benefit from the contribution of midwives.

Characteristics of government midwifery personnel

Ministers and policy-makers will require that the providers of a midwifery contribution to national policy have a comprehensive understanding of health, maternity and midwifery services, and can interpret midwifery in terms of national policy as well as being able to identify midwifery issues in the broadest sense. While the midwifery contribution should be supportive of the role of midwives as a resource for achieving successful outcomes to pregnancy, it should not promote or protect the profession for its own sake. The professional and personal experience and characteristics of midwifery personnel who work at ministerial or policy-making level are likely to include the following:

- wide experience in midwifery practice, probably at primary, secondary and tertiary levels;
- substantial experience at a senior level of management or education;
- broad knowledge and understanding of the maternity services and policy, and a knowledge of the wider health policies and services;
- experience of and ability to contribute to discussion and debate on health and maternity care at the local and national levels;
- good skills in oral and written communication; and
- good interpersonal skills, including the ability to facilitate effective working relationships.

Conclusion

This section has shown the need for and identified the elements of a midwifery function in health ministries or equivalent policy-making bodies. It has not dealt with the details of the role of midwifery personnel at this level, or the details of dealing with individual subjects and key issues. This task would arise once the principle of the midwifery function was established. It is hoped that the points put forward will generate discussion that will lead to the further strengthening of midwifery in support of safe childbirth in every country.

References

1. Splane, R.B. & Splane V.H. *Chief nursing officer positions in national ministries of health*. The Regents, University of California, 1994.
2. *Handbook of resolutions and decisions of the World Health Assembly and the Executive Board, Vol. III, 3rd ed. (1985–1992)*. Geneva, World Health Organization, 1993.
3. *European Conference on Nursing. Report on a WHO meeting*. Copenhagen, WHO Regional Office for Europe, 1989.
4. *Fourth Meeting of European Government Chief Nurses and Collaborating Centres for Nursing and Midwifery. Report on a WHO meeting*. Copenhagen, WHO Regional Office for Europe, 1995 (document EUR/ICP/NURS 94 03/MT04).

5. *Second Meeting of Government Chief Nurses of the Newly Independent States*. Copenhagen, WHO Regional Office for Europe, 1994 (document ICP/NURS 94 03/MT02).
6. *Moving more nurses into management positions*. Geneva, International Council of Nurses, 1991 (Press release No. 3).
7. *Challenges and opportunities: draft framework for action*. London, Commonwealth Secretariat, 1993.
8. Resolution WHA45.5 of the Forty-fifth World Health Assembly on strengthening nursing and midwifery in support of strategies for health for all. *In*: Salvage, J., ed. *Nursing in action. Strengthening nursing and midwifery to support health for all*. Copenhagen, WHO Regional Office for Europe, 1993 (WHO Regional Publications, European Series, No. 48).
9. *Mother–baby package: implementing safe motherhood in countries. A practical guide*. Geneva, World Health Organization, 1994 (document WHO/FHE/MSM/94.11).

6

"It ain't what you do; it's the way that you do it"

Adèle Beerling

INTRODUCTION

This chapter describes some of the work methods used by the staff of the Nursing and Midwifery unit of the WHO Regional Office for Europe. It is hoped that their experience may prove useful to other groups of nurses and midwives working for change in various settings. (Annexes 6–8 give specific tips on taking part in international meetings and small group meetings and raising funds.)

We who work in the Regional Office Nursing and Midwifery unit aim to help Europe's nurses optimize their contribution to achieving health for all. Given the widening gap in health status between countries in the European Region, action for nursing development is urgent; given the size of the task and the limited financial and human resources, the need for effectiveness is evident.

This chapter outlines our approach to achieving this aim. Notes on a participatory approach are followed by a discussion of the use of project management and notes on the motivation of our counterparts, especially those in CCEE and NIS. The chapter ends with a description of the role of networks and the special characteristics of our work environment. The old saw, "It ain't what you do; it's the way that you do it", indicates the importance of a well led process of change. The leading principle is that the process must be open and flexible, maintaining continuity but allowing for change and innovation as needed.

For illustration, many examples are taken from unit activities, particularly an education activity managed as a project. For a good understanding of the examples later in this chapter, a general introduction to this project is needed.

LEMON project

The LEarning Materials On Nursing (LEMON) project is designed to strengthen the contribution of nurses and midwives to health for all through education at all levels – formal and informal, basic and continuing. In the CCEE and NIS, and indeed in some other parts of the European Region, the lack of materials to support educational activities is a major obstacle to nursing development. Existing books, journals and guidelines tend to be outdated and difficult to obtain, and usually fail to address the needs of nurses and midwives.

In spring 1993, we therefore launched the LEMON project to provide a package of materials to all nurses and midwives in the CCEE and NIS (about 2.5 million people) in their own official languages. Groups in the countries have been involved from the start in selecting subjects and useful existing material and have reviewed all draft chapters, along with the international advisory group, which has members from eastern and western Europe. The short-term aim of the project is to make a core package of material available to as many nurses and midwives as possible; the long-term aim is for countries to become self-sufficient in selecting, writing and producing their own material. Capacity building is therefore an important parallel aim of the project and is supported by a collaborative structure and decentralized project management. The country LEMON groups are in charge of all aspects of project implementation, with support from the international network. In addition, the national and international project networks provide a good basis for future activities.

Support for Change

Since increasing nurses' contribution to health for all requires change, we looked at an approach to producing long-term change that appears increasingly effective in nursing practice: the normative–re-educative approach, as described in the WHO publication *Nursing in action (1)*. In this approach, change moves from the bottom up. It is based on the belief that people need to be involved in all aspects of changes that affect them, because they will accept and implement only the changes that fit their values, goals and relationships. This approach accepts the premise that people can best achieve change by acting collectively, with maximum involvement of everyone effected. Because the group owns the process and outcome of the changes, it is more likely to accept and sustain them. We use this approach in meeting preparation, networks and various forms of consultation. It is especially evident in the guidelines for developing a national action plan (see Chapter 4); team building and consultation form key steps in making an action plan that has a good chance of being implemented.

Example

A participatory style of work leads to meetings in which participation is facilitated as much as possible. The use of professional facilitators in the preparation and running of our meetings has proved invaluable. While the WHO organizers are concerned with the content of the meeting, the facilitators guide the participants through the process of the meeting. The aim is to make them feel comfortable in order to be able to participate fully, and to make the process of the meeting, the decision-making and the planning of activities open and visible. This makes the meeting a learning experience useful on other occasions. In short, a typical preparation process looks like this:

- determining the need for a meeting, in consultation with partners;
- setting dates and securing funding;
- inviting a small group of partners for a planning meeting led by facilitators;
- inviting feedback and input on the provisional agenda from the participants before the meeting proper; and
- conducting the meeting, led by the facilitators, with the participants at the small planning meeting acting as facilitators for group work, and acting as "eyes and ears" in general.

Meetings focus more on the sharing of participants' experience in plenary sessions and small groups, and less on lectures by experts from outside the group.

This method requires time, particularly in planning and preparation. We found, however, that the amount of time spent on preparation decreased as people came to know and trust each other and learned to value this way of working. We also found that people valued the time invested in preparatory activities, as well as the attention on process throughout meetings, as much as they valued other activities, such as the direct sharing of information.

Here is another example of investing in process and capacity building through a participatory approach. When holding meetings in the

CCEE and NIS, we pay attention to building up the organizing skills of our local counterparts. Although there are exceptions, many of them have had few opportunities to organize an international meeting; they can benefit from guidance in budgeting, negotiation, planning, and so on. This is time consuming, but local ownership of the meeting increases and often large savings are made on hotel and other expenses through creative and motivated input from the local organizers.

Taking a participatory approach is not always easy, especially when time is limited and the stakes are high for all involved. In practice, it means that a WHO initiative takes on a life of its own. We complete our role as initiator and catalyst, and our partners take over. This can be very satisfying from the point of view of sustainable development. A disadvantage is that this often makes our contribution to the end product difficult to distinguish, and WHO and its Nursing and Midwifery unit depend on visibility and recognition for their activities to gain further support, including funding.

Management Approaches

One chooses to organize an activity as a project. Some kinds of work benefit from this method; others certainly do not. To decide one must weigh up the advantages and disadvantages in comparison to other approaches. Project work, routine work and improvised work, are all used to tackle the tasks of the Nursing and Midwifery unit *(2)*.

Project work

With the project approach, one-off performances of high quality can be achieved with limited resources. To manage a project within an organization, existing tasks and responsibilities have to be reviewed and often replaced (partly or wholly) by a temporary structure. The problem to be solved or the situation to be achieved is defined in objectives. Progress to achieve these can be regularly reviewed. Activities have to take place in appropriate phases, which can make it impossible to use resources evenly.

Example

In the implementation phase of a project such as LEMON, many teachers are needed for the introduction of the package of learning materials. This causes a sudden peak in the need for training resources. Teachers play a role in the earlier stages that is far less substantial than that when they are actually giving workshops.

Routine work

This approach is preferable when a certain type of result has to be achieved regularly or several times, under similar circumstances and with similar resources available each time. The approach assists in delivering a product, service or activity of more or less the same quality regularly over a period of time. This often makes it easier to strive for efficiency.

An organization taking on a new activity or product as a matter of routine can keep existing tasks and responsibilities in place. If adjustments are necessary they should not disturb the existing structure. The problem to be solved is translated into a standard type of problem familiar to the organization, and outcomes can be predicted with reasonable certainty. The client who asked for the service, activity or product can leave the task with the organization; both partners know what will happen. All activities are spread as evenly as possible, permitting an even use of resources.

Example

We in the Nursing and Midwifery unit routinely provide information. We produce, review and distribute leaflets and other documents. We channel requests for information through a standard procedure, handing out document order forms to anyone requesting documentation. These forms are dealt with regularly and systematically, and stocks of documents are kept up to date. In addition, many service units in the Regional Office for Europe support us routinely, such as those for maintenance, supplies and the production and distribution of books and documents.

Improvised work

Improvised work provides an opportunity to respond flexibly to a new situation or a demand for a new product or activity. Action can start right after the problem presents itself, making it easier to strive for speed and flexibility. Existing procedures, rules and regulations are pushed aside; new rules are made up along the way. Ad hoc solutions are sought to bring fast and visible results. This approach, however, carries a risk of losing sight of the overall situation, of spending too much time in solving smaller parts of a problem and missing the connections between them. Quick action and a sudden burst of activity make the control of resources very difficult. We keep improvisation to a minimum, but it is unavoidable in some instances. Dealing with an unexpected visit from a close colleague or a sudden donation can be welcome grounds to improvise. Owing to the limited human and financial resources available to our Programme, we can seldom answer requests demanding an improvised approach.

Choosing an approach

The tasks of the Nursing and Midwifery unit vary, bringing different kinds of work needing different kinds of approach. Project management is a much used approach, combined with routine support for functions such as information provision. Improvisation takes place but we keep it to a minimum.

In project management, the aim and desired outcome are defined and the way to achieve them clearly signposted. Each signpost (or the initiation, definition, design, preparation, implementation and maintenance phases) provides an opportunity to review aims, to check on process and progress, and to make detailed plans for the next phase, thus providing a learning opportunity for all involved.

Example

The choice of a project approach for LEMON was based on the fact that the need for learning materials was urgent and required a unique solution. The aim and desired results were defined and could be reached by clearly defined steps; the resources and time-scale were reasonably defined and the project would be a one-off performance. The aim was to provide learning materials to meet the urgent need, but to do it in a way that built capacity in the participating countries to select and produce materials independently. It required an innovative approach that was both flexible and effective. The demand for learning materials was very clear. How WHO could meet this demand in a way that led to long-term benefit for the countries was a question that needed input from all involved. An advantage of the project approach is that it gives plenty of opportunity for both learning and participation. A participatory approach is valued for its motivational function; partners feel they are involved in and have ownership of the project.

One way of answering the urgent need for learning materials could have been to raise funds for the mass transfer of western materials. We dismissed this approach for several reasons. It would lead to dependence on learning materials from sources outside the user countries and would not stimulate local production. Such material would always reflect the situation in the country it was written for, leaving little room for the independent assessment and development of nursing in a user country.

The LEMON project has developed a package of materials with the participation of the future users, combining selected existing materials with new items produced for the purpose, and choosing a format that allows user countries to adapt the package to their local needs. In this way, the package comes as close as possible to answering the need for learning materials, as it is compiled by experienced and knowledgeable partners from the user countries. At the same time, the participatory approach creates a learning process for everyone involved, which includes teaching participants about assessing needs, setting priorities and making decisions.

The project partners valued this learning opportunity. One of them said that even if they had never had the actual LEMON package, the project would still have been a success. It had made them discuss the problem and take their own actions.

Motivation and its Relation to Working Methods

Why do people invest energy in making changes when social, political and economic circumstances make their own professional and personal lives so complex? More concretely, where can a nurse in central Asia find motivation for change when her salary has not been paid for months and was not enough to keep her family fed in the first place?

Sources of motivation

We have met many dedicated colleagues who are committed to nursing development. Wondering what motivated them to start working with us and, later, to continue their engagement, we identified some facts and made some assumptions. The facts are that:

- the health ministries in countries are formally committed to achieving health for all;
- the cost–effectiveness of health care services needs to be increased;
- nurse leaders in countries repeatedly expressed the need for nursing and midwifery development through education; and
- faced with the needs of a patient or client, most professional nurses want to be able to provide the best possible care.

Facing these facts, we have assumed that:

- decision-makers in ministries are willing to invest in the development of nursing because of its cost–effectiveness and its potential contribution to specific health outcomes; and
- the desire to provide the best possible care results in a willingness in some health workers to invest time and energy in action leading to nursing development.

This being so, we use motivation as part of our approach.

The LEMON project and all our other activities require input from the participating countries. Often this boils down to individuals or small groups making a personal investment in getting the job done. One reason for such an investment is that the activity strongly relates to what participants have already done or wish to do, since the activity was initiated after consultation and collective assessment of needs and priorities. This makes our activity not an additional task, but part of the participants' existing tasks, although it may require a different approach from what they would normally choose.

Another motivating factor is visible results. In most of the countries participating in LEMON, social, political and economic changes have created instability in people's lives. A new leader brings new ideas, new plans. Many new plans are not carried out before another changeover comes, making it difficult to see progress and believe that a vision and plans lead to concrete results. In our nursing and midwifery activities, of a vision for the future of nursing, strategic planning exercises (national action plans) and practical, visible action have proved to be a powerful combination.

Example

Our workshops on the development of national action plans for nursing (as described in Chapter 4) and our international meetings of government chief nurses often include the preparation of meeting statements (Annexes 1–4). These are visible results of the meetings, in which the next concrete steps to be taken by all parties directly after the meeting are agreed. Such statements facilitate action among both participants and the colleagues and other interested people to whom the statements are sent.

Education is often identified as a key issue for nursing development in country workshops on national action plan development. An introduction to the LEMON project then becomes a logical part of the workshop, giving the participants opportunities for immediate action while continuing the development of a national action plan.

Rewards

People are often motivated to do a job because it brings them money, which gives them access to what they want. Partners in our nursing and midwifery activities receive no money other than what they earn in their jobs as health workers or administrators. In parts of the European Region it is not uncommon that salaries are not paid for months. Health service salaries are often very low and not enough to support a family.

These circumstances force many people, including some of the most talented and experienced, to seek other employment. Our partners mention the following rewards from their involvement with our activities:

- a positive feeling about involvement with an international organization in general, and WHO in particular;
- a higher personal profile resulting from involvement in nursing development and international work;
- opportunities to meet like-minded colleagues and build relationships with colleagues in other countries; and
- opportunities to learn from activities in their own and other countries.

Examples – international activities
The value ascribed to participation in an international meeting arises in part from the associated benefits, including the opportunity to network and to see other countries. Participants at our meetings know that the work is intensive and requires a lot of energy. Every minute of a meeting is used. In addition, the language of our meetings is either English or Russian, so most participants must communicate in a language other than their mother tongue, which is extremely tiring, especially after long and often uncomfortable travel. Furthermore, the agendas are full and the number of days available for a meeting is restricted by everyone's workload and the expenses. To accommodate the desires for both networking and sightseeing, however, we schedule long coffee and lunch breaks for networking whenever possible, breaks in the afternoon for sightseeing and evening sessions to get as much work done as possible. Often the host country generously offers hospitality in beautiful places.

LEMON sends out a monthly newsletter called *LEMON news* with contributions from LEMON country groups, the international advisory group and the WHO Nursing and Midwifery unit. Among other things, the newsletter is a monthly reminder and proof of the readers' international involvement.

Example – working with like-minded colleagues
Becoming part of a subgroup, a group that works together for a common goal, can be valuable. People can deal with daily frustrations more easily when they know they are part of a group that shares these frustrations and tries to make changes for the better. Sharing a problem can unite people in action. It can also be a legitimate way for people to spend work or leisure time on activities that really interest them.

Many LEMON groups in countries have divided their tasks among subgroups. This means that some subgroups have worked for around two years on particular topics, such as fund-raising or publicity, and have built up considerable experience. This can widen the scope of the participants' regular jobs.

Example – participatory approach
Although cultures in countries vary tremendously, many seem to value a participatory style of management *(3)*, a conclusion also reached by external evaluators of our work.

Shared decision-making is very important in our programme and in its work with partners. This means that our partners are informed about the issues, and have a chance to reflect on, talk about and form an opinion on them. In the end decisions are made, often by consensus, rarely by WHO decree.

Example – competition
Once people are involved in nursing development, competition can be a motivating factor. This can mean competition with the activities of other groups, such as nursing associations or councils; or competition with other countries taking part in activities initiated by WHO. Progress is valued, and well implemented activities and visible results are a source of pride to the participants.

Many country LEMON groups are strong in publicizing the project. This gives a higher profile to nursing in the countries and wins increased support for the project. In addition, group members gain inspiration and motivation from comparing their efforts and sharing their ideas with colleagues from other countries.

Example – momentum
In times of social, political and economic change, people can take the opportunity to ride the wave of change and pursue their goals more effectively in temporary disarray. Our partners say that now is their chance to make the changes.

Example – results
Finally, involvement in our activities brings results for nursing development in countries, through both the content of activities and the methods used to carry them out. A participatory style and the attention paid to building skills in leadership, strategic thinking and programme management build capacity for the future. The process side of our activities offers learning opportunities for everyone involved. The knowledge and skills acquired in the implementation of an activity can be applied to many situations in work and life.

As mentioned, the facilitators of workshops for government chief nurses help to develop the leadership skills of the participants, particularly those used in taking part in a meeting, working in a group, reporting, increasing self-awareness and creating peer support.

For the translation of the LEMON package, intensive discussions took place in the countries to select the correct current expressions for new nursing concepts. Often no words were available in a given language, and new ones had to be found. In other words, as a result of the LEMON project, the professional language in many countries has expanded. This provides important support to other nursing developments.

Flows in motivation

Naturally, the level of one's motivation varies. Our priorities in work and life in general change over time; new commitments can replace older ones. In addition, some activities are more appealing than others and people's tastes vary. To continue a valuable activity when key people decide to step aside, we must plan for this eventuality from the start. In all our activities, we value both the essential contribution of established, experienced and respected colleagues and the enthusiasm and energy of new colleagues. The new partners' possible lack of experience and knowledge can easily be balanced by their new ways of looking at issues, new techniques and new contacts with another generation of nurses and midwives. Furthermore, partners are sometimes required to step aside; political changes in countries often replace the staff in ministries and therefore our counterparts.

Example

In establishing a group of leaders for the development of a national action plan for nursing or a country group for LEMON, we encourage our partners to value each other for their specific skills and to recognize that workloads are heavy for most and that other priorities may arise. Although for practical reasons we encourage groups to have no more than 10–15 members, we also encourage them to look for other partners who can carry out parts of the tasks, and continuously to consider new talent. In national and international meetings, we encourage new people to participate on a small scale so they can be gradually integrated into the work. Of course, this is easier said than done: delegating tasks in the project in which one feels deeply involved is difficult; letting go and making room for others often require will-power and self-control. Adding new members to a well functioning group often slows the pace of the work and causes distrust and tension.

NETWORKS AND THEIR ROLE

We commit much of our time and other resources to the development and maintenance of networks. They are essential because they provide us with information on the kind of activities needed, and they are a vehicle for implementation. We need such a vehicle because resources are too limited to reach directly all the people whom our networks now reach. In addition, good networks build the capacity to solve problems. By creating and maintaining networks, we invest in the development of tools to enable nurses to solve problems for themselves. Finally, networks are key elements for the implementation of the kind of activity that we can offer.

With the limited resources available, we must concentrate on what WHO and our programme can do uniquely or better than other organizations operating in the same field. From the nursing viewpoint this unique role focuses primarily on the following *(4)*:

- support for long-term, sustainable development, especially through promoting the implementation of sound policies and guidelines;
- the development of national policies for nursing and midwifery within the framework of strategies for health for all;
- drawing nurses from the CCEE and NIS into the international community through networks and WHO collaborating centres; and
- producing and recommending high-quality written materials based on the principles of health for all and other WHO policies.

Nurses or others in governments who are responsible for nursing, are our key partners, alongside the collaborating centres and LEMON networks. No other organization can or is attempting to create a pan-European network of government chief nurses, who should be leaders of nursing reform within the framework of health care reform and advocates within their own ministries, as well as entry points for all other activities.

The findings of Gaye Heathcote *(5)* appear to be applicable to our networks. She divides the functions of networks broadly in two: professional development and social and moral support. Professional development needs typically include:

- the sharing and development of skills, particularly in problem solving, group work and communication, and facilitation and negotiation;
- the updating of information on current issues of concern; and
- the sharing of experience and expertise, particularly in relation to effective methods and passing on useful tips.

Social needs typically include:

- maintaining social contact with people in a similar work situation;
- providing and receiving moral support to help in one's daily work; and
- interacting with colleagues in a nurturing and supportive social environment.

The ways in which these professional and social needs are articulated and responded to vary according to the channels of communication, the participants' knowledge of the needs and the resources available to the group. The WHO network of European government chief nurses depends very much for its maintenance on the meetings organized by the Nursing and Midwifery unit, the news that we disseminate and individual contact between network members. Obstacles to intensive and regular contacts include the geographical distances between members and the sometimes limited access to means of communication such as telephone, telefax and electronic mail. Our networks fulfil the needs outlined by Heathcote; on numerous occasions, members have supported each other and cooperated on activities outside the scope of the network. Lack of time and financial resources, however, regularly hampers the maintenance of the networks.

The conditions identified by Heathcote *(5)* as essential for initiating and maintaining effective networks include:

- careful consideration of the timing and location of meetings;
- an agenda set well in advance, that has been collectively discussed and agreed by the group as a whole;
- a structured, developmental approach to professional growth that includes a variety of methods and resources;
- formal recognition of the network at the national level;
- a dynamic, non-authoritarian and participatory management style that overtly values and rewards each individual's contribution; and
- rotation of the facilitator role, with an organizational team being seen as more desirable than vesting responsibility in one person.

Our leadership role in network meetings includes coordination and is seen as a valuable resource, but it also acknowledges every participant's role as an expert during the meeting and subsequent activities.

To maintain a network, one should ensure that mechanisms that promote both continuity and change are built into its characteristic processes and procedures. The continuity of our networks depends very much on the resources available; those available in the past (especially voluntary donations) have allowed regular meetings once every one or two years. Despite the relatively long time between meetings, the members are increasingly familiar with each other. As a result, they need less time to renew their acquaintance at the start of a meeting, and they make decisions more swiftly because they value each other's opinions.

Another important factor in maintaining a network is its flexibility; it must be responsive to changes such as new members, conditions and priorities. Skilful facilitation allows feedback and criticism to be used constructively and modifications to be implemented without any loss of confidence in the network itself. In addition, the network must look critically at its own performance to be able to learn and grow. This is essential for the partners in our networks, since their time and finances are so limited that they must be spent particularly wisely.

Our meetings have a participation rate close to 100%; this underlines the importance of the networks. Again, the participatory approach, including the interchange of roles, is seen as a valuable strategy because it can capitalize on individual members' strengths, expertise and experience. It is also part of creating a caring and supportive environment for carrying out the functions of the network. In evaluating the meetings, members of our networks repeatedly stress the value they ascribe to this method.

Characteristics of Effective Multicultural Cooperation

In its work for nursing development, an international organization such as WHO has much in common with other organizations, but also has special characteristics and conditions of work. Like many other organizations, WHO must cope with reduced budgets and increased need for cost–effectiveness with reorganization as just one of the areas for attention. Because WHO is an international organization, many cultures meet in the work of the nursing and midwifery programme. As noted by Wendy Griswold *(3)*, multiple cultures are always potentially cultures in conflict. Both in the programme and in our relations with partners, we work in a multicultural environment. Research has identified a number of basic elements or variables common to all cultures around which communication is built *(6)*. Recognizing differences in these variables is a starting point for an effective intercultural communicator. Dodd *(7)* cites the following:

- cultural roots
- cultural personality
- material culture
- economic organization
- roles and culture
- kinship relationships
- political organization
- social control
- art
- language
- stability
- cultural belief system.

It is beyond the scope of this chapter to expand further on these variables, but they illustrate the complexity of cooperative work in the multicultural setting of WHO. Griswold *(3)* notes that organizations that operate in more than one country or involve several cultural groups in a single country face the complex situation of different people and organizations having their own ideas and values that may not be understandable or mean the same to others. Although managers cannot change the fact that those differences exist, they can recognize the lack of control and take action to plan and work with those differences.

This further strengthens the case for a participatory approach to planning and implementation; in multicultural work, direct communication, shared decision-making, respect for all partners and the potential for capacity building are particularly valuable. The approach is also important in relation to another basic factor in our work: the fact that most of our partners are women with all the characteristics that arise from women's position in society. Empowering women, increasing their role in decision-making and helping them take charge of the changes that affect their professional lives are essential to long-term sustainable change.

Conclusion

While concentrating on what the WHO Nursing and Midwifery unit can do uniquely or better than others, we promote a strong participatory approach to the process of change in nursing. Project management, as well as other forms of management, are used. Our guiding principle remains our openness and willingness to change, guided by the demands of the ever-changing social, political and economic environments in the Member States of the WHO European Region. We value the process of change as much as the content of nursing development, and are careful to create a working environment in which everyone involved can learn, be empowered and progress.

References

1. Salvage, J., ed. *Nursing in action. Strengthening nursing and midwifery to support health for all.* Copenhagen, WHO Regional Office for Europe, 1993 (WHO Regional Publications, European Series, No. 48).
2. Wijnen, G. et al. *Working in projects*. Heerlen, Spectrum, 1988.
3. Griswold, G. *Cultures and societies in a changing world.* Beverly Hills, CA, Sage Publications, 1994.
4. *Evaluation of the EUROHEALTH programme.* Copenhagen, WHO Regional Office for Europe, 1994, pp. 1–50 (document EUR/RC44/BD/1).
5. Heathcote, G. *Networks, their role in the professional development and support of health educators*. London, Health Education Authority, 1991.
6. Egorenkova, Y. *Achieving peak performance in a challenging international environment; a communication strategy for the Nursing and Midwifery unit.* Copenhagen, WHO Regional Office for Europe, 1993 (document).
7. Dodd, C.H. Dynamics of intercultural communication. Dubuques, 1982.

Part III
Work in Progress

7

The role of nursing in primary health care

Sally Campbell

This chapter takes the form of a discussion paper on the development of nursing roles in PHC. It is aimed at nurses at all levels and in all areas of the profession and at personnel with roles allied to nursing, such as health service managers, doctors, support workers or health care assistants. The chapter is intended to contribute to the design, delivery and strengthening of public health policies and health care services.

The first recommendation from the 1988 WHO European Conference on Nursing *(1)* in Vienna states that: "All nurses ... should be strong advocates for policies and programmes for health for all at national, regional and local levels". The call from WHO for nurses to play a key role in achieving health for all and the positive response from nurses make it important that nurses be able to identify the nature of that role and what is involved in carrying it out.

The activities of the nursing and midwifery programme of the WHO Regional Office for Europe are designed to help nurses respond to the profound changes in health care in the European Region and to meet the challenges of the strategy for health of all *(2)*. The programme aims to help nurses acquire the necessary leadership skills to play a full role in health policy development at all levels, and to develop nursing practice that focuses on health and the reduction of inequalities in health.

As identified at the Vienna Conference, this means that nurses need to develop innovative services based on a PHC approach that focuses on health rather than disease. This reorientation will particularly challenge the nurses who work in community settings, and so this chapter focuses on this area. Nevertheless, a refocusing on health and the reduction of inequalities in health are essential for all nurses, wherever they work.

Nurses need to develop new knowledge, skills and attitudes to do this. All must base their work on a clear and holistic understanding of the concept of health. Nurses need to learn more about what causes inequalities in people's health status, and to recognize them as politically, economically and professionally unacceptable and a common concern to the whole profession. If nurses view health as a basic human right, they need to ask why some people are denied this right, and why health inequalities persist in the countries of the European Region *(3)*.

This chapter begins by placing nursing in its wider context by examining the overall strategy of PHC, including the continuing relevance of the health for all movement and the importance of working with communities and developing team approaches. It goes on to examine the role of the nurse in PHC and the evidence that nursing care does indeed benefit the individuals, families and communities that come into contact with it. Innovative examples are given to demonstrate the potential of nursing work in PHC. Finally, the chapter considers how the challenges of the future may be taken up. It discusses the need for clear aims and definitions of nursing in PHC, and examines the reasons for the pressing need for the further development of nursing roles in PHC, along with appropriate educational preparation.

As shown in Part I of this book, the title of nurse and its associated roles and functions vary enormously. Titles, roles, places of practice and educational preparation show great diversity in the WHO European Region alone. This chapter is aimed at personnel in occupations related to nursing, which includes feldshers and midwives. The inclusive term nurse is used purely for ease.

This chapter does not aim to provide a definitive text on nursing in PHC, so it does not discuss each and every nursing role found in every country. The variations across the Region are immense, and change is occurring so rapidly that information quickly becomes obsolete.

At present the European Region has 50 Member States. As in Part I, for clarity and ease, they have been divided into three groups: the CCEE, the NIS and the so-called western European countries. Obviously, differences occur within each group; where possible and applicable, these differences are noted. There can be no guarantee of accuracy in the statistics used, as change in countries is rapid and statistics may be lacking, inaccurate or subject to adjustment.

The Strategy of PHC

The foundations of health

WHO's definition of health – a state of complete physical, mental and social wellbeing and not merely the absence of disease or infirmity – is possibly the most widely used in existence. It has been criticized for its apparent assumption that health cannot exist if a person has a disease or infirmity, but it was intended to purvey a sense of holism, the recognition that health is made up of physical, mental and social factors. This first definition has since been developed to encompass the concept of health as being the ability to adapt to change and to realize one's potential. This is expressed in a 1984 statement *(4)* that defined health as:

> the extent to which an individual or group is able … to realize aspirations and satisfy needs; and … to change or cope with the environment. Health is … seen as a resource for everyday life, not the objective of living; it is a positive concept emphasizing social and personal resources, as well as physical capacities.

The statement recognizes that health is a dynamic state and that each person's potential is different. The notion of health as the foundation for achieving human potential deserves consideration by health care workers. In this sense, health promotion becomes the empowering of people to become all they are capable of becoming; it is linked closely with improving people's quality of life and it is an individual and societal responsibility *(5)*.

The foundations of health comprise the basic needs of food, drink, shelter and warmth. In many countries of the European Region, these foundations have yet to be attained. For example, 110 million people (about 12% of the Region's population) still lack access to safe drinking-water *(6)*. In many countries, food shortages make an adequate diet impossible, and displaced and homeless persons lack shelter and warmth.

A wider definition of health includes education to obtain information about factors that influence health. The concept of community is important: a person is never completely isolated, so his or her actions may have a significant influence on others in the community. The individualist philosophy within the political structure of some countries promotes the notion that people are solely responsible for their health. This results in a victim-blaming position on health and detracts from the need for social, economic and political action to achieve a healthy community.

The influences on health are diverse and easier to describe than health itself. This fact may make it hard to identify the primary targets in work for health, and certainly people's and countries' needs are diverse. Nevertheless, a comprehensive multisectoral approach to health is essential if these basic needs are to be met. The collective approaches to health laid down in the Declaration of Alma-Ata *(7)* and the Ottawa Charter for Health Promotion *(8)* recognize this fact; they promote the idea of PHC.

Health for all through PHC

The Declaration of Alma-Ata *(7)* reaffirmed WHO's original definition of health, and emphasized that health should be considered a fundamental human right. Since then, the health for all strategy has fostered a worldwide movement to reduce disparities in health and bring about change in the way health is perceived, promoted, protected and created. The Declaration aims to influence government development plans and local research agendas and action plans. In 1991, the original European targets for health for all were revised, retaining their framework and direction but adding the new priorities that the Region requires *(2)*. Six major themes underpin the targets:

- equity is the essence of health for all;
- the promotion of health and the prevention of disease are important strategic issues in the policy;
- people themselves will achieve health for all;
- many sectors of society must collaborate in order to achieve the goal;
- a harmonious health system focuses on PHC and adequate referral services, and provides affordable, high-quality care; and
- an increasing number of health problems transcend national frontiers and require international action.

The WHO health policy for Europe consists of 38 targets that list improvements in health status expected over the next 20 years, and the changes in lifestyle, the improvements in the environment and the developments in prevention, treatment, care and rehabilitation that are necessary to attain the targets, along with the policy formulation, support and coordination necessary to implement these approaches *(2)*. The policy acknowledges that global inequities in health are not primarily medical but political.

The need to focus health services on PHC is seen as the key to attaining the primary goal: the attainment by all people of the world of a level of health that will permit them to lead socially and economically productive lives. PHC can be defined as *(7)*:

> essential health care based on practical, scientifically sound and socially acceptable methods and technology made universally accessible to individuals and families in the community through their full participation and at a cost that the community and country can afford to maintain at every stage of their development in the spirit of self-reliance and self-determination.

PHC is essential care available to everyone and easily accessible from homes and workplaces. It gives people the information they need to gain control over their lives and health. It treats common diseases before they get worse. It also implies the universal involvement of the population in determining its own needs. PHC could act as a catalyst to involve community groups in care. The information function includes distributing information within the health care system, sharing it with the users of services and providing it to the general public. Another function is to reach out to emerging priority groups in society, including ethnic minorities and migrants, children, the homeless, unemployed people, and those dependent on drugs or at risk of contracting AIDS. Advocacy is an important function, and includes both helping service users to speak for themselves about their needs and speaking for the health sector. All of these could be said to contribute to the function of empowerment: enabling people to take charge of their own health. Empowerment is a function of increasing importance, but requires knowledgeable PHC teams and service users to succeed.

PHC should be the foundation for services and constitute the first element of a continuing health care process. Health care should focus on locally accessible PHC, supported by secondary and tertiary care that is comprehensive and responsive to health needs. A wide range of services for health promotion, disease prevention and cure, rehabilitation and support should be available to meet the needs of the population, and special attention should be given to the needs of high-risk, vulnerable and underserved people and groups. The PHC strategy of promoting decentralization and community participation is designed to reorient health policy to meet the needs of disadvantaged groups in society. Indicators of progress could be determined centrally and locally, combining national planning with local self-determination. Within this framework, some communities may well see some of the disease-oriented approaches to health care as relevant but within a context that puts the goals of creating strong communities first *(9)*.

The Declaration of Alma-Ata advocates the adoption of PHC as the means to achieve health for all *(7)*. This ideal is widely accepted, yet change is slow in coming. Governments are reluctant to invest resources in PHC because the long-term benefits are difficult to demonstrate in a limited amount of time; instead, they favour measures that are quick in delivering results, such as the high-technology care in specialized hospitals. The dominance by the medical profession of health care services, and its demand for high status, high salaries and high technology has helped to perpetuate this situation. The PHC ideal needs to be rejuvenated if a new world view of health and a new strategy for the delivery of health care are to be realized.

Effective PHC requires cooperation and coordination among health professionals, individuals, families and community groups. How can people tackle these issues when a great many live and work in societies where the opinions of the population are not sought and paternalistic relationships between health professionals and their patients are common? How can people facilitate team spirit in PHC? The following section explores the issues of community work and the concept of the PHC team.

Working with communities

The Vienna Declaration *(1)* highlights the importance of promoting the active involvement of the community in setting health care goals. The focus is shifting away from treating individuals towards building relationships with families and communities, and this is reflected in the targets for health for all *(2)*. The targets give a framework in which nurses can achieve their traditional aims in new, more independent ways, in close collaboration with other health professionals, their clients and communities.

The WHO approach to PHC emphasizes the role of community participation in the promotion of health. This means that local people identify their needs and professionals act as resources to enable and facilitate empowerment and the redistribution of power. The goal is to improve health status with the powerful combination of professional skills and the people themselves. Community groups and networks that involve health care workers can be established to increase partnership and the power to bring about change. For this to work, policies and plans need to be publicized and recommendations invited, so the community's expressed needs are taken into account in the planning of services.

The Community Mothers Programme in Ireland *(10)* is an example of nurses enabling true community participation. It is a support programme for first- and second-time parents who have children aged 0–2 years and live in areas of social and economic disadvantage. It aims to give power to parents by developing their parenting skills and building confidence and self-esteem, so that they tackle their problems in their own way.

The key resource of the Programme is the 150 community mothers. They are experienced mothers who have raised children in the participating communities. They visit young mothers at home to give them support, encouragement, and advice and information on health care. The Programme acknowledges the parents as the experts in the care of their children. The work is based on giving information for change, rather than advice and instructions on how to raise children. The community mothers are trained, monitored and guided by family development nurses with a background in public health.

An evaluation of the Programme reveals that its objectives are being met. The parenting skills of young mothers in deprived areas are being enhanced through community participation. The community mothers feel they have benefited from the programme through self-development and increased self-esteem and the family development nurses have gained an insight into the lives of families living in poverty and deprivation; this assists them in developing appropriate programmes to improve the health of the population. This simple and effective programme at grass-roots level is a great example of how health status can be improved by mobilizing existing resources, in this case experienced mothers, with little expenditure and no high technology.

The fostering of community action and health promoting approaches to care enables health professionals to shift their focus from sickness to wellness. Raising awareness of certain issues in communities and encouraging people to take action allows them to wield more social and political influence. Nevertheless, one must accept that health professionals and communities often have different priorities, and a balance must be struck. In addition, community action cannot solve all the causes of poor health; it can make a contribution, but should not detract from the political solutions to problems.

This approach to community work encourages the concept of teamwork and partnership among health professionals, individuals, families and community groups. The goal of teamwork is to improve health status with the powerful combination of professional skills and the people themselves. Health professionals must be able to pull together in equal relationships to improve their work. The following section looks at the issues surrounding teamwork.

The importance of teamwork

The PHC team brings together the different skills that a patient or client needs, and combines them in a way not possible to individual workers *(11)*.

In western European countries, the term PHC usually describes what is more accurately called general medical practice. The PHC service offered to patients is centred around the general medical practitioner and the work is usually seen as having a curative orientation *(12)*. The demographic changes in European populations, however, mean that health needs to be seen in a wider perspective, as an integral part of social and economic relationships.

The responsibility for health should be transferred from the doctor, as a healer, to a PHC worker, as a partner *(13)*. Cooperation between health professionals is essential. In the United States, studies have demonstrated that collaborative practice between nurses and doctors results in care that is equal to or better than the care provided by doctors alone *(14)*.

Achieving this cooperation requires the PHC team to shift its focus from medical care to health care. No single health profession can provide all the services required for good, comprehensive PHC. A multidisciplinary team is necessary to meet the many and varying needs of the population it serves. The PHC team may be made up of people who share a common purpose, but this alone is not enough to ensure a successful working relationship *(15)*. Some of the characteristics of successful teams have been described as follows *(16)*:

- the team consists of a group of identified people;
- the team has a purpose and objectives that are known to and agreed on by all members;
- members are selected because they have relevant expertise;
- members know and agree on their own roles and know those of the other members;
- members support each other in achieving their common purpose;
- members trust each other, and communicate with each other in an open, honest way; and
- the team has a leader whose authority is accepted by all members.

The size of the team may affect its ability to work effectively; there should be enough people to be creative and innovative and yet allow space for everyone to contribute. A team of at least 2 and no more than 15 people allows this kind of exchange to take place. Regular team meetings facilitate communication and cooperation; at such meetings aims and objectives can be set, support and advice provided and the relationships between professional colleagues developed. The team pools knowledge, skills and resources, and shares the responsibility for the final outcome of its decisions. The fact that people may all work in the same building does not in itself create a team. The team that chooses common goals and encourages the discussion and monitoring of successes and failures is more likely to thrive.

The development of protocols or guidelines for use by the PHC team may facilitate the move towards collaborative care. A protocol may be defined as an agreement to a particular sequence of activities that assists the health care worker to respond consistently in complex areas of clinical practice. The protocols developed by the team may improve teamwork and consequently client care. A collective approach to this development encourages the sharing of expertise and knowledge, and enables the process of auditing clinical care. It may not be possible to develop protocols for all situations that health professionals face in the course of their work. There are large areas of uncertainty in the management of many conditions. The team should recognize this by not treating protocols as law, and avoiding protocols where the scientific evidence is not sufficient to support their use. Professionals should use protocols as guidelines to good care, but individualize the care where necessary and recognize that accountability rests with them, not the protocols. Protocols may then be used as the basis for standard setting and evaluation of the effectiveness of work.

Audit and evaluation are important tools for assessing the PHC team's work. Audit is self-review or peer review, often involving an examination of records and discussion of individual cases *(17)*. Evaluation requires making a judgement about the value of something; it is the process of assessing what has been achieved and how. It means looking critically at an activity or programme, working out what was good about it and what was bad, and how it could be improved.

People may make evaluations to improve their practice, build on their successes and learn from their failures. They may use the findings to help other people improve their practice and avoiding repeating others' failures. Evaluation may also be used to justify the allocation of resources to the work, and to provide evidence to support the case for continuing it. Evaluation can give people the satisfaction of knowing how useful and effective their work has been, and to identify any unplanned or unexpected outcomes that could be important.

Donabedian *(18)* identified three aspects of health care that are amenable to evaluation: structure, process and outcome. Structure includes the resources, facilities and organizational settings; process comprises the set of activities that go on between practitioners and patients, and outcome is the change in a patient's current and future health status that can be attributed to the health care they have received. Outcomes are the ultimate validators of effectiveness and the quality of care, but process is important, too. It includes the interpersonal aspects of care that are of considerable concern to patients and are likely to affect the outcome *(19)*.

Measuring outcomes can be a difficult problem. Perhaps changes in health awareness can be assessed by measuring the interest shown by consumers or monitoring changes in demand for services. Changes in knowledge or attitude can be assessed by observing changes in what clients say and do, or by conducting interviews and discussions between health care providers and clients *(16)*. Nevertheless, how does one measure the effectiveness of care for arthritis sufferers, which is unlikely to have an easily definable end-point, or a child with otitis media, where the condition is likely to be self-limiting? Patients and doctors or nurses may differ in the objectives that they consider important.

Teamwork on such tasks as standard setting and evaluation is more easily achieved when team members function well together. Each should be treated as and feel like an equal of the others, although all must accept the leader's authority. The latter may be difficult in a situation where no one person is responsible for the coordination of family care. PHC provision is often split into specific areas of practice, such as adult and paediatric care, obstetrics and gynaecology. The increasing decentralization of decision-making and financial responsibility in health care in many countries increases the importance of leadership and management skills for all categories of staff. The team needs to be able to translate its common purpose into specific performance goals. Common objectives centred on the patient are likely to be more successful.

Training programmes should reflect the need for collaboration between the different disciplines involved in PHC. Practical training in developing teamwork could focus on the characteristics of successful teams, helping people to identify their teams' needs and problems. Training shared between different professional disciplines improves communication and teamworking skills.

Teamwork means shared decision-making, overlapping roles and attention to the processes through which a group works. A system that undervalues some members prevents meaningful teamwork from taking place. Collaboration and teamwork can be strengthened when members work closely together; professionals whose work is based at the same site have more opportunity to build successful working relations through formal and informal contact. This contact can be further improved by shared client or patient records. Furthermore, multidisciplinary education helps to ensure that team members understand their roles and professional responsibilities.

Nursing in PHC

The tradition of nursing

It is useful at this point to look briefly at the tradition and value of nursing. Health care has developed at various levels in different parts of Europe, and consequently today's care givers vary widely *(3)*. The development of nurses and midwives into an educated and professional group has varied greatly from country to country, but in general has three main branches: care of the sick, midwifery, and public health nursing or preventive care. Nursing has evolved within the traditional pattern of caring for and curing others. The care of women in childbirth is part of this tradition. Nursing is therefore seen as a fundamental human activity.

As described in Part I of this book, nurses and midwives now comprise the largest single group of health professionals in the European Region, at present numbering around five million. Yet nursing has been constrained from reaching its potential in countries all over the world for several reasons.

The first is a theme shared internationally: the fact that most nurses are women. Nurses in all countries inherit a legacy of underdevelopment, domination by the medical profession and gender discrimination. Nursing shares the characteristics of other female-dominated occupations – low pay, low status, poor working conditions, few prospects for promotion and poor education *(20)*.

This fact is compounded by the confusion over the meaning of the title nurse. In many countries the title is not protected by legislation, so it may be used not only by people with degrees in nursing but also by those who have completed only brief task-oriented training for the role. In some regions unqualified health care assistants may not call themselves nurses but their dress is the same, making it difficult for patients to distinguish between qualified and unqualified staff.

Furthermore, health care in the modern world has developed into a largely curative system, alongside advances in medicine. As medicine developed, the role of the nurse was extended to include helping doctors to use medical technology. Nursing education and training became dominated by medicine, with doctors assuming powerful roles in teaching, examining and regulating nurses, as well as defining their role. In many countries this is still the case. Nursing work turned into delegated medical tasks and the fundamental caring activity was eroded *(3)*. Curricula have concentrated on the tasks of nursing, which has led to professionals who often work in a task-oriented way. In many countries, basic nursing training contains little or nothing on how to provide health education to patients.

Much of nurses' work today reflects a profession that has carved out its role around these constraining forces. The subordination of nurses, first to doctors and now to nurse managers, has hindered participation in planning PHC services for patients. Consequently, nurses have found their work restricted by the illness-focused models of medical practice. Many aspects of the work carried out and the decision-making responsibilities of the nurse are invisible, avoiding any conflict or challenge to the medical profession *(21)*. For example, a nurse explained that she acted as a clerical assistant when the doctor was on duty, but was required to do his work after he went home. The problem with this situation is that the true abilities of the nurse go unrecognized and unacknowledged. Things are little better in rural areas; the nurse may be recognized as the only health professional available to give care, but this is of no consequence because the system does not value PHC and resources are concentrated in the hospital. Such conditions perpetuate the low status and value of nursing in the community.

In the former USSR, clever children were trained to become doctors, and the reward for being a very good nurse was often admittance to a medical school. This system means that nursing is not valued as a profession in its own right. It also prevents successful nurses from acting as role models for their colleagues. The prestige of nursing is low; in a recent survey only 26% of nurses stated that they would choose to remain in nursing if another choice were available to them *(22)*. A further effect of low status and salary is that it is impossible for nurses to be healthy themselves; the study showed that nurses are unlikely to spend their leisure time in active pursuits; few have the chance to leave their town, 50% did no physical sport, and nearly 70% spent their last holiday at home. In addition, 18.4% cited their health as poor, and 69.3% as only average *(22)*. Without the recognition they deserve, nurses cannot have the skills, knowledge and enthusiasm needed to participate in the initiatives identified in the targets for health for all.

Tradition has defined a good nurse as being a good woman. This has been both a strength and a weakness of the profession. The tradition of the relative unimportance, low status and pay and poor conditions of women's work has undoubtedly been the weakness. However, the strength is that nursing has always been associated with a caring environment rather than a curative one *(23)*. The increasing number of elderly people living with chronic ill health and the growing failure to match the demand for medical services with available economic resources mean that creating a caring environment is increasingly seen as the way to provide PHC in the future. Nurses are, therefore, at the forefront of this future approach to health care.

The Vienna Declaration *(1)* clearly defines nursing as being concerned with achieving and maintaining health; it focuses on the person, and not a disease state. In areas of practice such as health assessment, counselling and preventive health care, research has shown that nurses are at least as skilled as doctors, if not more so *(24)*. A study of general practice in the United Kingdom found that the nurse was able to provide safe and effective care of hypertensive patients, and had more success in areas of preventive care such as obesity *(25)*. In the United States, nurse practitioners have successfully demonstrated that they can provide first-contact PHC as safely and effectively, with as much satisfaction to patients, as a family doctor *(26)*. The literature review by Feldman et al. *(27)* shows that nurse practitioners working in primary and ambulatory care settings are valued by their patients, and able to provide good care with improved access. They are a potential source of lower-cost care and likely to spend more time with patients.

In the United Kingdom, a review of existing research by the Audit Commission *(28)* and the Centre for Health Economics at York University *(29)* has demonstrated a direct correlation between the employment of qualified nurses and better patient outcomes. Another study *(30)* demonstrated that work by nurse practitioners is diverse, associated with a high degree of patient satisfaction, and focused on wellbeing as well as illness. It also found nurse practitioners to practise safely and effectively and to generate savings in some areas. Numerous studies *(26,31,32)* have shown that appropriately educated nurses and midwives give care of comparable quality to the services provided by doctors at a much lower cost. Nurses and midwives are particularly effective in providing services for prevention and those depending on communication with patients. Determining value for money requires the consideration of cost and quality, and nurses score on both accounts *(33)*:

> The data are accumulating to attest to the powerful contribution nurses are making to enhance the quality of care, promoting health and lowering total system costs. Nursing is a bargain in and out of hospitals. We need to make the results of these studies available to policy makers.

The examples given here of nursing studies in the United Kingdom and the United States demonstrate how nurses can increase health gain, give care that is equitable, accessible, cost-effective and appropriate, and empower their clients. This is not to say that nursing in the CCEE and NIS should mimic that in the rest of Europe or the United States. Aims and objectives necessarily differ; obtaining clean water and sanitation or the means to carry out an immunization programme (rather than a complex screening programme) may be the goals of community nursing in some regions. Nurse managers must base care on the health needs and participation of the population with which they work. Health care can be effective only if it is inseparably linked to the environment in which people lead their daily lives.

The almost five million nurses in the European Region represent a critical mass that can have positive influences on the population's health if its potential is realized. The PHC model is a powerful one and the prospect of nurses as a force of caregivers – economically viable, professionally equipped and technically able – is attractive. One way of realizing the potential of the nurse is to develop the role through experimentation in the field, using the patient as the focus.

The following section looks at examples of innovative practice. The first describes the introduction of a new nursing role to the existing health care system, and the second illustrates a long-established health worker role with great potential for development. The examples outline how the principal components of PHC may be incorporated into the role of nursing in the future.

The section title uses the word examples with reason. The word model may suggest the adoption of the roles presented, but these examples are included to illustrate the innovative ways of caring that nurses have developed in their own environments. Transplanting a role to a different health care system is unlikely to work because of the differing influences on health, illness and health care. The influence of nurses from the west is strong, and some assume that western medicine is required to improve the health of the people in other regions of the world. Consequently, as nurses have shared their models and theories, nursing education has taken on increasingly uniform attitudes and beliefs *(34)*.

Exposed to transplanted attitudes and beliefs, many nurses have experienced a confusion of values. For example, Minami *(35)* argues that Japanese nurses rarely question the underlying values and beliefs that are represented in the models and theories developed in the United States. Western views of independence, autonomy, individualism, freedom, rights, obligations and democracy have been transmitted to Japanese nurses, even though Japanese values can be very different. Newly graduated nurses in Japan find that a conflict of values arises when they try to put into practice the ideas that have developed during their education. Minami *(35)* argues that Japanese nurses should retain traditional values and evaluate their effect on professional nursing practice. This demonstrates the need for the development of indigenous and traditional modes of care rather than the adoption of practice from very different systems.

Examples of Innovative Practice

The nurse practitioner

The role of the nurse practitioner has recently emerged in British PHC in response to perceived inadequacies in the provision of health care services. It comprises advanced practice by professional nurses, whose additional knowledge, skills and attitudes enable them to assume responsibility for health assessment and the management and delivery of services at the first level of a health care system *(36)*. The nurse practitioner's responsibility is essentially the provision of PHC, involving individual and family care, community and programme development, case-finding and health education. In addition, nurse practitioners have shown themselves to be capable of assuming responsibility for the diagnosis and treatment of common problems and providing continuity of care at the local level *(37)*.

The concept of the nurse practitioner began in 1965 in Colorado, in the United States. It was a direct response to the shortage of appropriately qualified doctors in some rural and urban areas, resulting in gaps in health care. The nurse practitioner role and a pilot programme of study were developed to meet this need *(38)*. Since then, the role has flourished and more than 25 000 registered nurse practitioners are working in all areas of health care in the United States. Nurse practitioners perform a comprehensive range of activities that greatly expand nursing practice, as well as replacing some of the work previously done by doctors. Much research on the role in the United States amply demonstrates its benefits to patients, with regard to health promotion and maintenance and increased compliance with treatment regimes *(39)*.

In the United Kingdom, interest in the development of nursing roles in PHC has been growing over the last 5–10 years. Government reports and subsequent health reforms have advocated increasing the scope of practice of nurses working in PHC *(40)*. In response, the Royal College of Nursing embarked on the first diploma programme for the preparation of nurse practitioners in 1990; the programme is now offered at the level of a first university degree. The students are required to be experienced practitioners, as the course aims to build on and extend what they already know. A sound educational base for practice is vital, as this will allow the nurse practitioner greater scope of practice while safeguarding the safety and efficacy of the care offered. Educational preparation includes gaining knowledge and skill in interviewing and history taking and physical nursing skills, including examination and assessment, recognizing abnormalities and screening clients for disease risk factors and early signs of illness. The students gain clinical experience in their places of work, where they acquire skills in physical examination, problem solving and the diagnosis of patient problems through close facilitation by a GP. In addition, this fosters close working relationships with supportive medical colleagues in the workplace. Subsequent research has shown that nurse practitioners working in close collaborative relationships with doctors are able to use their skills comprehensively and effectively *(30).*

The Royal College of Nursing has developed a role definition and *modus operandi* for nurse practitioners *(41);* here is how the role is defined:

> A nurse practitioner in primary health care offers direct access to clients seeking health care. She is able to undertake initial assessments of any health problems likely to be encountered in a primary health care setting, and, following assessment, can initiate treatments falling within her range of knowledge and skills. The nurse practitioner can admit people to the primary health care system, both by offering initial treatment herself, and by referral to others, including physicians.
>
> The nurse practitioner evaluates the effectiveness of treatment she has carried out at suitable intervals, and, when appropriate, will discharge her clients from the primary health care system.
>
> As a practitioner of nursing, she will offer an educational, supportive setting for clients to explore their health problems, and will work with them for as long as necessary, enabling them to regain health.

The *modus operandi* comprises the following *(41)*:

> The nurse practitioner in primary health care settings practises an expanded nursing role and makes professionally autonomous decisions for which she has sole responsibility. She receives clients with undifferentiated undiagnosed problems, diagnoses and prescribes treatment as well as providing

> care herself. She works closely with other members of the primary health care services, respecting professional role boundaries and acting in the best interests of clients.
>
> The nurse practitioner may practise independently, or within an organisation, and will exercise a right to refer or admit clients to the appropriate services and resources. These include other professionals by referral, and an agreed range of services.

This provides a framework from which to practise, but it is recognized that nurse practitioners' flexibility is their strength and that rigid role boundaries should be avoided. Nurse practitioners are most effective when they can practise across a range of settings, wherever the care is needed, rather than being restricted to one area *(42*). The practitioner is therefore likely to cross several boundaries between health professions in the community, particularly with regard to prescribing drugs for treatment. This area of practice is usually seen as the preserve of the medical profession, but is under review. Legislation was recently changed to allow certain nurses to prescribe from a limited drug formulary. This new approach to health care aims at providing a service to its users that is responsive, efficient and effective *(43)*.

The nurse practitioner's focus of care is the client, not the disease and its cure; this gives assessment and treatment a broad base, with room for the nonmedical aspects of disease, such as the planning of long-term care or rehabilitation, along with the consideration of the social and emotional effects of illness *(37)*. The first large research study of nurse practitioners in the United Kingdom found that the patients expressed a high rate of satisfaction with the care provided, apparently because they valued the practitioner's consultation style *(30)*. This was said to be wide ranging and social, rather than only medical and technical. Importantly, the nurse practitioners were all found to be practising safely and effectively. Consultations were usually found to be longer with a nurse practitioner than with a GP, although nurses working in a close partnership with GPs were found to have shorter consultation times, fewer referrals and greater cost savings than those in outreach work. This finding was also affected by the relative experience of the nurse practitioner; the more experienced had correspondingly shorter consultation times and fewer referrals *(30)*.

The role of the nurse practitioner would appear to be an appropriate model on which to build empowering health care for clients *(43)*. Stilwell et al. *(44)* demonstrated that, although nurse practitioners dealt with patients presenting problems, they were also concerned with long-term preventive strategies, such as measuring blood pressure or taking cervical smears when appropriate. Listening and providing health education were important components of consultations. Salisbury & Tettersell *(25)* found that a nurse practitioner using agreed protocols provided equal or better care than doctors in the management of hypertension and obesity.

The accountability and responsibility of nurse practitioners for patient care are crucial to the success of their role. This is a new concept for nurses, who have traditionally been protected from responsibility by nurse managers and doctors, but one that needs to be taken up if they are to develop an autonomous role. The legal framework for practice can either support or limit the opportunity for broader and more extended responsibility for PHC nursing. For example, in 1992 the United Kingdom's governing body for nursing, the United Kingdom Central Council for Nursing, Midwifery and Health Visiting, produced a document called *The scope of professional practice (45)*. This provides a framework for nursing practice, reflecting the personal responsibility and accountability of individual practitioners. It explicitly states that the nurse should work only within her or his level of competence and skill. The document enables practitioners to make decisions about their own boundaries of professional practice. This approach to the regulation of nursing is broad enough greatly to facilitate the development of nursing roles in the United Kingdom while protecting the public.

Lack of coverage and difficulty in access to services are just two areas in which nurse practitioners have been found to make a difference. In the United States, nurse practitioners have brought good quality PHC to rural districts where there are no medical practitioners *(39)*. In the United Kingdom, nurse practitioners have demonstrated their ability to provide complementary health care alongside the doctor, and care to people who lack access to the system, such as the homeless *(46)*. The health care gap differs in every community, but nurse practitioners have great potential to meet the PHC needs of the local population. Their holistic and autonomous approach to practice frees them from many of the previous constraints on nursing.

The feldsher

The role of the nurse practitioner shares some similarities with that of the feldsher. While the latter had its origins in the PHC system of the former USSR, it is still widely practised in the CCEE and NIS.

The feldsher's role in PHC is that of an additional health worker, and is viewed as falling somewhere between nursing and medicine. Indeed, there was some discussion about giving the feldshers the title of deputy doctor, but this did not happen. The feldsher is an autonomous practitioner who can provide basic treatment, care and preventive services. The work comprises elements of medicine, nursing, public health and community development. An important and positive point is that feldshers usually return to their home towns or villages after training and are therefore an integral part of the communities they serve. The role and training of feldshers in the CCEE and NIS are described in Chapter 2 (see pp. 60–62).

Many rural areas lack doctors, and care is provided by feldsher/midwife posts or stations, which provide PHC to local people. The units generally consist of one feldsher, one midwife and one nurse. In some of the urban units, a doctor has a visiting role; visits can be sporadic, however, for several reasons, including high workload or difficulty in obtaining fuel for transport.

Feldshers provide community care, including home visits, and are usually senior to nurses. They are able to provide health assessments and diagnostic and therapeutic care, to perform examinations and tests, to recommend treatment plans and to prescribe some medication. Feldshers can also refer patients to doctors at rural ambulatory units and central district hospitals. They also work in emergency services and in occupational health. Preventive care is said to be an important aspect of feldsher training.

Many feldshers work in units or from their homes, with very limited access to the resources they need to provide good services. Disinfectants, medication and vaccines are in short supply; often there is no sterilizing equipment and disposable items are used several times. In Kazakstan, it is estimated that more than 50% of feldsher/midwife stations have no telephones *(47)*. Nurses and feldshers may have to walk to their patients and spend valuable time searching and queuing for medicines and fuel. In remote rural areas, these health professionals take responsibility for their patients' welfare with very little support from other professionals or the infrastructure.

An example of innovative practice is found in Uzbekistan, where the Red Cross has teamed up with local feldsher/midwife stations to improve health care. The Red Cross found the feldsher/midwife station an extremely valuable and successful model of care that needed resources to operate efficiently. The Red Cross, feldshers and nurses carried out some research to establish a basic package of care for the users of the service. This included information about nutrition, water and hygiene, medication and the equipment needed in a feldsher/midwife station. The Red Cross was then able to provide each unit with a bed, basic sterilizing equipment, instruments for medical procedures and medication. It also provided instruction to nurses and feldshers in further skills, and the use and maintenance of the equipment.

Feldsher training is usually separate from nurse education, although it takes place in the same medical schools. It emphasizes health education and the prevention of ill health. Several branches of specialist feldsher practice exist, such as the feldsher midwife, whose responsibility is maternal and child health. The sanitary feldsher participates in the control and monitoring of environmental concerns, such as clean water, and the control of epidemics. The stomatology feldsher is trained to assist the dentist.

Nurse and feldsher training encounter many practical difficulties, as described in Chapter 2. Because professionals have difficulty in obtaining continuing education, their practice is based on tradition. Some aspects of practice have been proved to be detrimental to the health of the patients, such as the tight swaddling of newborn infants. Teaching is often theoretical with no clinical supervision in the practice environment.

These difficulties are partly the reason why many of the CCEE are discontinuing feldsher training. Underfunding and neglect of PHC services has led to difficulty in recruiting or educating appropriate staff, so the role is inadequately performed. People seem to have forgotten that feldsher/midwife stations have tried to give whole populations access to health care under extremely difficult conditions.

The association of the feldsher role with the old Soviet system is another reason for its decline in popularity. The attraction of the western world, with its individualist policies, privatized health care and high medical technology, is powerful. In some countries, the whole health care budget is given to secondary care in hospitals, so no funding is available for PHC. Feldshers and nurses working in the community have been forced to leave their jobs because their salaries have not been paid, leaving many of them without any health care.

Nevertheless, training for felshers continues in the central Asian republics, where these personnel are widely acknowledged to be a vital part of the PHC team if health care is to be offered to a very scattered population, often living in difficult terrain. In addition, the use of feldshers is seen as a more economical solution than attempting to increase the numbers of doctors in practice.

The countries that are discontinuing feldsher training run the risk of dismantling the old system before a new one is in place, and losing many of the good qualities of the feldsher role in the race towards western-style health care. In some areas, feldshers are the only health workers who can act autonomously and provide a package of care to the community. Health care reform must be based on the needs of the people and the countries' resources. It is useful to remember that the planners of health care in the United States are also attempting reform because their own health services have become exclusive and technology driven, at the expense of the health of the lower socioeconomic strata, where most morbidity occurs.

The Way Forward

The key concept for the future development of nursing is the need to create a nursing role that is appropriate to people's health needs, rather than the needs of the health care system. Nurses need to base their work on the five principal components of PHC reiterated by the WHO Expert Committee on Nursing Practice *(48)*:

(a) universal coverage of the population, with care provided according to need
(b) promotive, preventive, curative and rehabilitative services
(c) effective, culturally acceptable, affordable and manageable services
(d) involvement of the community in the development of services so as to promote self-reliance and reduce dependence
(e) approaches to health that relate to other sectors that contribute to development.

The entire nursing infrastructure – from basic nursing education to development in practice, management and leadership – needs to change if nurses, feldshers and midwives are to take up the challenge of PHC. Nurses need to recognize their contribution to the promotion of health in the primary care setting and challenge the dominance of one form of knowledge over another *(49)*. In addition, the attitudes of other health professionals need to change if nurses are to take up their role as equal partners on the PHC team. As long as nursing continues to be undervalued, nurses will be unable to make a worthwhile contribution to health care planning and services.

The same fundamental problems are being experienced all over the world *(50):* there are too few primary care providers and too many specialist care providers, and health personnel are concentrated in urban areas and prefer to train in clinical specialties rather than in public health, health policy and management *(50).* The providers of health care must shape the service that they offer their patients and clients if they are to own ideas and innovations. Such ownership is necessary for the commitment needed to ensure good quality care. This need should not be underestimated; caring requires the caregiver to make an emotional investment. Without this commitment, good care is impossible to achieve. The emotional labour of caring is particularly difficult where conditions of work are poor. Low status, low pay, poor working conditions and long hours demoralize any workforce. Unfortunately, these factors are common and can lead to the loss of ability to provide care. How can nurses inspire good quality care and innovative approaches when they have no textbooks written for them in their language, no equipment to use, no proper place from which to practise and no support from other health professionals? Countries across Europe must develop career structures and incentives if they are to encourage nurses to move into generalist roles in PHC in underserved areas.

This time of dramatic change offers the unique opportunity to reshape nursing's place in health care, so that nurses are more closely allied with the needs of the patient rather than the medical profession *(22).* Nurses in PHC are in an ideal position to empower the patient through their equality of relationships and their willingness for partnership with their patients. Change often occurs first in the field, with policy reform following. This means that clinical professionals and their clients often bring about the first changes, with policy-makers following. For this reason, the number of nurses leading and managing PHC teams needs to be increased, and nurses should have greater responsibility for making decisions within health care teams *(48).* Clients' opinions need to be sought and the environment needs to be right if change for the better is to occur. This will result in a service that is responsive to both the individual and the collective needs of its users.

Nursing has responded to the needs of the patient by developing different models of care, but these have not been developed in a systematic way. Today, nursing can be difficult to define and differentiate from the roles of other health care workers. For nurses to take up an equal membership on the PHC team, a clear definition of their role needs to be established.

A clear definition of the role of nursing will also help to establish the appropriateness and usefulness of its role in PHC. A definition that broadly describes nursing in terms of aims and goals, rather than specific tasks, will help to clarify what nursing is and consequently what direction its development should take. A WHO publication *(20)* supports the 1988 Vienna Declaration *(1)* and gives a clear outline of what nursing comprises:

> nursing … is to help individuals, families and groups to determine and achieve their physical, mental and social potential, and to do so within the challenging context of the environment in which they live and work. This requires nurses to develop and perform functions that promote and maintain health as well as prevent ill health. Nursing also includes the planning and giving of care during illness and rehabilitation, and encompasses the physical, mental and social aspects of life as they affect health, illness, disability and dying.
>
> Nurses ensure the active involvement of the individual and his or her family, friends, social group and community as appropriate in all aspects of health care, thus encouraging self-reliance and self-determination …
>
> Nursing is both an art and a science that requires the understanding and application of the knowledge and skills specific to the discipline. It draws on knowledge and techniques derived from the humanities and the physical, social, medical and biological sciences.
>
> The nurse accepts responsibility for and exercises the requisite authority in the direct provision of nursing care. She is an autonomous practitioner accountable for the care she provides. She has a responsibility to assess her personal needs for continuing education in management, clinical practice and research, and to take action to meet those needs.

This broad description clearly sets out the nursing role without imposing yet more constraints. A definition needs to be dynamic if nurses are to promote evolutionary nursing practice; nursing needs to be able to grow with the changing health care needs of society. Flexibility is needed if PHC is to be responsive to the needs of service users, so the lack of a rigid definition is a strength at a time of rapid growth in medical knowledge and technology. Medical and nursing practice is becoming more complex and the traditional boundaries between the professions are being pushed back. The boundaries of health care work often shift, and doctors are used to passing on some of the routine parts of their work to nurses. A little blurring around the edges of roles can allow the transference of tasks to more suitable professionals without arousing the territoriality so often apparent in doctor–nurse relationships. A less definite demarcation of roles in PHC benefits the patient, as practitioners can use their experience, education and skills to meet changing needs for care. This is clearly a positive step towards the empowerment of the professions and the people they serve.

If interprofessional teamwork is to succeed, and nurses are to realize their potential in full, they and their medical colleagues must change the stereotypes of their roles, and nurses must take part in decision-making at all levels. The development of an autonomous practitioner role in the community would be a positive step. Autonomy entails the right of self-government and freedom of will. It is not the same as independence. Total independence from the medical profession is not necessary or desirable, but nurses must be allowed to use their clinical experience and judgement to shape the scope of their role in PHC in order to provide appropriate care to their clients. A good example is the recent development of a hospital of nursing care in Kazakstan. Patients who are elderly or have cancer or physical disabilities are cared for in a hospice environment. Nurses run and staff the hospital, using their expertise to provide appropriate care.

Education is a key to developing excellence in nursing practice. Basic programmes of nursing education with a strong emphasis on PHC are needed to produce generalist nurses able to function in both the hospital and community. The health needs and the social and economic circumstances of each country should form the basis of curriculum development, to enable the profession to respond to current and future health problems in PHC. The decision to shift the focus of the basic nursing curriculum to PHC usually comes from the highest level of government. Ministries of health and education, and legislative and regulatory bodies, need to consider training in the light of the number, types and quality required of the different categories of health care worker. If nurses are to achieve clinical effectiveness, the right numbers of qualified and experienced nurses are needed, with their expertise recognized and utilized.

The nursing curriculum should be reformed to ensure that health professionals learn about the philosophy of health development as defined in the Declaration of Alma-Ata *(7)* and the global strategy for health for all *(51)*. The curriculum needs to emphasize assisting and enabling people to meet their own health needs, fostering the maintenance and promotion of health, and providing health education along with care in the community. This view is supported by research; for example, a project in Norway *(52)* revealed that community nurses needed to know more about nursing in the home setting, particularly what type of help local authorities offer to clients, and how to help clients gain access to it. The researchers recommended that demographic changes and increasing knowledge about the process of aging be reflected in training. Nursing education should include knowledge of the care of the elderly, which should include the pathology associated with aging as well as methods and models for working with elderly patients. More elderly clients use the health services, and they have more chronic illnesses and compound problems than any other group in the general population. Nurses need competence in rehabilitation, preventive medicine and cooperation with different professional groups and departments and patients' families. This example demonstrates the need for a clear link between practice and education.

At present, the education of most health professionals is firmly based in an individualist philosophy that focuses on treating bodies *(53)*. Most learning of health care practice takes place in specialized, institutional settings rather than at the primary and community levels, and rarely with any involvement of the users of services in identifying their needs. Exposure to the primary and community settings would increase the relevance of the education given to health professionals.

The community is the nurse's largest and most complex client in PHC. Nurse educators need to teach not only the traditional roles of caring for individuals and families in the community but also how to nurse the community as a whole. Students need experience in the community to acquire skills in community-based assessment and programme development. They need to learn more about the theory and practice of community development work, such as those that guide the practice of public health nursing *(51)*. The specialist knowledge and skills subsequently acquired should rest on this foundation. Education in advanced practice should include a knowledge of epidemiology, biostatistics, health services administration, public health policy and the use of personal and group influence to bring about change *(13)*. The question of when and how to specialize in nursing is difficult to answer in all parts of the Region; local circumstances must guide development. A clear, achievable action plan for each country and PHC team is needed to inform these decisions.

Basic training needs to include wider issues, such as how to teach the basics of hygiene to a community, how to support women making choices about fertility control or how to promote breastfeeding to young mothers. Importantly, nurses often need such information for themselves, and this can be a great motivation for learning and sharing with others. For example, in Kazakstan abortion continues to be the most common form of family planning, with the average woman having five abortions in her lifetime. A small study of 416 nurses in Kazakstan *(47)* revealed that over 33% of those surveyed did not know what family planning was, and only 38% could cite different methods of contraception.

Nurses need to identify their learning needs and expectations; such opportunities are rare in many places at present. In the former USSR, task-oriented training given to quite young people made this approach impossible. It is hoped that change will come through schemes such as the WHO LEMON project (see Chapter 6), whose long-term aim is for the countries involved to become self-sufficient in selecting and writing their own learning materials. The move to greater professional autonomy in nursing through control of the educational experience offered to students will lead to a dynamic change in the approach to nursing. Nurses will no longer be uncritical practitioners, merely following others' orders. They will become critical thinkers, reflective practitioners, able to offer and be accountable for patient-centred care *(55)*.

Education to develop research skills and the tools of evaluation will facilitate nurses' ability to examine their practice, see what is effective and develop their practice accordingly. Research will lead to the development of the profession in the PHC field. If nurses are not properly educated and prepared, practice becomes unresponsive to experience and research, particularly if another professional group controls the educational process and uses it for its own benefit *(55)*. The new approach to learning and professional development should result in an increase in professional competence *(56)*. Nurses' reflection on themselves, their situation and their understanding – that is, reflection in action – will make professional practice more effective *(57)*. Nursing education needs to abandon the task-oriented approach and promote inquiring minds.

Basic training needs to be reoriented, and the concept of learning as a lifelong process needs to be adopted. Access to postbasic education in nursing improves nursing care and the motivation and retention of staff. Integrating teaching and practice ensures that teaching is relevant to practice, and brings high-quality nursing practice to the health care system *(58)*. Nurses who have opportunities to advance their practice through education become valuable PHC workers who can take up roles in the community. Nurses whose experience and expertise are underpinned by research-based knowledge have the ability to widen their scope of practice, strengthen their decision-making skills and become more independent and autonomous in practice.

CONCLUSION

As mentioned, the nursing profession makes up the largest single group of health care workers in the WHO European Region. In many countries and settings, nurses are the first, last and most consistent points of contact that people have with the health care system. The care offered by nurses has a significant impact on the population's health. If nurses are to be effective and efficient, the right numbers of qualified and experienced personnel need to be available and their expertise needs to recognized and utilized *(59)*.

Nursing practice within a PHC framework takes place in hospitals, clinics and communities. Hospital nursing should not be abandoned, but its emphasis should be reduced in favour of services and health promotion efforts where people live and work *(13)*. The nurse's practice should focus on improving people's health by working alongside the patient or community, and with other relevant health professionals. Achieving these changes requires a fundamental transformation of nurses' role as medical assistants to doctors; they must be well educated professionals whose unique and distinctive contribution to health care is respected by all colleagues, and who are regarded as equal partners in the health care team.

If the countries of the European Region are to achieve the targets for health for all *(2)*, they need to mobilize their health care workforce. Nurses – as economically viable, professionally equipped and technically able caregivers – present an attractive prospect. Appropriate education, research and nursing roles are necessary to reach this ideal. Supportive legislation and regulation are needed to allow nurses to fulfil their potential and practise comprehensively where most needed. The issues of low pay, poor working conditions and low status need to be addressed. The development of career structures and incentives will encourage the movement of nurses into generalist roles in PHC.

The need for relevant research is clear; evidence-based practice enables progress in the scope and practice of nursing. Relevant education, however, is needed in virtually all countries of the Region, so that nurses can utilize research findings and carry out their own projects. This chapter has cited the evidence from existing research that nursing care benefits individuals, families and communities. Demonstration projects are needed to bridge the current gap between the theoretical concept of PHC and its implementation. This need is especially great in developed countries that possess complex health care systems primarily dedicated to cure and rehabilitation. In nursing research, achieving health for all provides a framework in which nursing theory could be developed, tested and evaluated. The community would become a partner in the expansion of nursing knowledge *(54)*.

References

1. *European Conference on Nursing. Report on a WHO meeting.* Copenhagen, WHO Regional Office for Europe, 1989.
2. *Health for all targets. The health policy for Europe.* Copenhagen, WHO Regional Office for Europe, 1993 (European Health for All Series, No. 4).
3. BARRETT, K. Life, health and the environment. *In*: *LEMON package.* Copenhagen, WHO Regional Office for Europe, 1995 (document).
4. NUTBEAM, D., ED. *Health promotion: a discussion document on the concepts and principles.* Copenhagen, WHO Regional Office for Europe, 1986 (document).
5. SEEDHOUSE, D. *Health: The foundations for achievement.* Chichester, John Wiley & Sons, 1986.
6. *Health in Europe.* Copenhagen, WHO Regional Office for Europe, 1994 (WHO Regional Publications, European Series, No. 56).
7. *Alma-Ata 1978*: *primary health care.* Geneva, World Health Organization, 1978 ("Health for All" Series, No. 1).
8. Ottawa Charter for Health Promotion. *Health promotion*, **1**(4): iii-v (1986).
9. BAUM, F. & SAUNDERS, D. Can health promotion and primary health care achieve health for all without a return to their more radical agenda? *Health promotion international*, **10**(2): 149–160 (1995).
10. *Community Mothers Programme. Evaluation report.* Dublin, Eastern Health Board, 1994.
11. ØVRETVEIT, J. Team decision-making. *Journal of interprofessional care*, **9**(1): 41–51 (1995).
12. *The contributions of family doctors/general practitioners to health for all.* Copenhagen, WHO Regional Office for Europe, 1991 (document EUR/ICP/PHC 348).
13. BARNES, D. ET AL. Primary health care and primary care: a confusion of philosophies. *Nursing outlook*, **43**(1): 7–16 (1995).
14. SOX, H.C. Quality of patient care by nurse practitioners and physicians: a ten-year perspective. *Annals of internal medicine*, **91**(3): 459–468 (1979).
15. LAMB, G.S. Two explanations of nurse practitioner interactions and participatory decision making with physicians. *Research in nursing and health*, **14**: 379–386 (1991).
16. EWLES, L. & SIMNETT, I. *Promoting health: a practical guide*, 2nd ed. London, Scutari Press, 1992.
17. GABE, J. ET AL., ED. *The sociology of the health service.* London, Routledge, 1991.
18. DONABEDIAN, A. *Explorations and quality assessment and monitoring. Vol. 1. The definition of quality and approaches to its assessment.* Ann Arbor, MI, Health Administration Press, 1980.

19. *Nursing beyond the year 2000. Report of a WHO Study Group.* Geneva, World Health Organization, 1994 (WHO Technical Report Series, No. 842).
20. SALVAGE, J., ED. *Nursing in action. Strengthening nursing and midwifery to support health for all.* Copenhagen, WHO Regional Office for Europe, 1993 (WHO Regional Publications, European Series, No. 48).
21. STEIN, L.I. ET AL. Sounding board: the doctor–nurse game revisited. *New England journal of medicine*, **322**(8): 546–549 (1990).
22. KARAGULOVA, J. & ASIMOVA, G. *Brief report of research work performed by WHO centre on primary health care and nursing on the theme: improvement of health manpower resources management in provision of primary health care programme.* Almaty, WHO collaborating centre on PHC and nursing, 1994 (document).
23. OAKLEY, A. What price professionalism? The importance of being a nurse. *Nursing times*, **80**(50): 24–27 (1984).
24. MOLDE, S. & DIERS, D. Nurse practitioner research: selected literature review and research agenda. *Nursing research*, **43**(6): 362–367 (1985).
25. SALISBURY, C.J. & TETTERSELL, M.J. Comparison of the work of a nurse practitioner with that of a general practitioner. *Journal of the Royal College of General Practitioners*, **38**: 314–316 (1988).
26. SPITZER, W.O. ET AL. The Burlington randomized trial of the nurse practitioner. *New England journal of medicine*, **290**(5): 251–256 (1974).
27. FELDMAN, M.J. ET AL. Studies of nurse practitioner effectiveness. *Nursing research*, **36**(5): 303–308 (1987).
28. AUDIT COMMISSION. *The virtue of patients: making best use of ward nursing resources*. London, H.M. Stationery Office, 1991.
29. CARR-HILL, R. ET AL. *Skill mix and the effectiveness of nursing care.* York, Centre for Health Economics, University of York, 1992.
30. NHS EXECUTIVE SOUTH THAMES. *Evaluation of nurse practitioner pilot projects. Summary report.* London, Touche Ross & Co., 1994.
31. SHI, L. ET AL. A rural–urban comparative study of nonphysician providers in community and migrant health centres., **109**(6): 809–815 (1994).
32. OFFICE OF TECHNOLOGY ASSESSMENT. *Nurse practitioners, physician assistants and certified nurse–midwives: a policy analysis, health technology case study.* Washington, DC, US Government Printing Office, 1986 (OTA Publication No. 37).
33. AIKEN, L. & FAGIN, C. *Charting nursing's future: agenda for the 1990s.* Philadelphia, PA, Lippincott, 1992.
34. PARFITT, B. The need for a universal definition of nursing. *Health care analysis*, **3**: 52–60 (1995).

35. MINAMI, H. East meets West: some ethical considerations. *International journal of nursing studies*, **22**(4): 311–318 (1985).
36. SALVAGE, J., ED. *Nurse practitioners: working for change in primary health care nursing.* London, King's Fund Centre, 1991.
37. BOWLING, A. & STILWELL, B., ED. *The nurse in family practice: practice nurses and nurse practitioners in primary health care.* London, Scutari Press, 1988.
38. BLISS, A.A. & COHEN, E.D. *The new health professionals: nurse practitioners and physician assistants.* Germantown, MD, Aspen Systems Corporation, 1977.
39. VENTURA, M. Assessing the effectiveness of nurse practitioners. *Nursing times*, **84**(9): 50–51 (1988).
40. *Neighbourhood nursing – a focus for care.* London, H.M. Stationery Office, 1986.
41. INSTITUTE OF ADVANCED NURSING EDUCATION. *Nurse practitioner diploma curriculum development document.* London, Royal College of Nursing, 1992.
42. CASTLEDINE, G. *The role and function of clinical nurse specialists.* Thesis, University of Manchester, 1982.
43. RIVETT, G. Comment. *In*: Salvage, J., ed. *Nurse practitioners: working for change in primary health care nursing.* London, King's Fund Centre, 1991, pp. 74–79.
44. STILWELL, B. ET AL. A nurse practitioner in general practice: working style and pattern of consultations. *Journal of the Royal College of General Practitioners*, **37**: 154–157 (1987).
45. *The scope of professional practice.* London, United Kingdom Central Council for Nursing, Midwifery and Health Visiting, 1992.
46. BURKE-MASTERS, B. The autonomous nurse practitioner: an answer to a chronic problem of primary care. *Lancet*, **1**: 1266 (1986).
47. KARAGULOVA, J. & ASIMOVA, G. *More effective to train nurses as a force in primary health care.* Almaty, WHO collaborating centre on PHC and nursing, 1993 (document).
48. *Nursing practice. Report of a WHO Expert Committee.* Geneva, World Health Organization, 1996 (WHO Technical Report Series, No. 860).
49. STREET, A. *From image to action: reflection in nursing practice.* Geelong, Victoria, Deakin University Express, 1991.
50. NEUFELD, V. ET AL. *Leadership for change in the education of health professionals.* Maastricht, Network Publications, 1995.
51. *Global strategy for health for all by the year 2000.* Geneva, World Health Organization, 1981 ("Health for All" Series, No. 3).

52. SOLHEIM, M. The need to develop the level of competence of auxiliary and state-registered nurses working in home care service. *In: The contribution of nursing research: past–present–future. Proceedings of the 7th Biennial Conference of the Workgroup of European Nurse Researchers (WENR), Oslo, Norway, 3–6 July 1994*. Oslo, Workgroup of European Nurse Researchers, 1994,vol. 2, pp. 901–915.
53. TURNER, B. *Medical power and social knowledge.* London, Sage, 1987.
54. JOLLEY, M. & BRYKCZYNSKA, G., ED. *Nursing care: the challenge to change*. London, Edward Arnold, 1992.
55. FORD, P. & WALSH, M. *New rituals for old: nursing through the looking glass*. Oxford, Butterworth and Heinemann, 1994.
56. STILWELL, B. *Nursing practice in today's world: a background paper*. Geneva, World Health Organization, 1995 (document).
57. ROGERS, R., ED. Bibliography and useful information. *In*: *LEMON package*. Copenhagen, WHO Regional Office for Europe, 1995 (document).
58. *Glossary of terms used in the "Health for All" Series No. 1–8*. Geneva, World Health Organization, 1984 ("Health for All" Series, No. 9).
59. CLARK, J. Expert nursing: A necessary extravagance. *European journal of cancer care*, **4**: 109–117 (1995).

8

Measuring nursing

Gunnar H. Nielsen

MEASURING NURSING AND DEVELOPMENTS IN NURSING

The emergence of an international classification for nursing practice, the continuous development of clinical quality in nursing and the growing use of electronic patient records for the documentation of nursing practice are three important recent developments that are linked in different ways to the issue of measuring nursing.

In medicine, the history of the International Statistical Classification of Diseases and Related Health Problems, whose tenth revision (ICD-10) was recently issued by WHO *(1)*, dates back to the eighteenth century. The history of an international classification for nursing practice began in 1989, when the ICN decided to supplement existing international classifications of medical diagnoses and procedures by developing a classification of nursing problems or diagnoses, interventions and outcomes *(2)*. This initiative is thus not conceived as a classification of nursing tasks, in the narrow sense of the word, but as a contribution to the existing family of health-related classifications that describe both the health status of the patient or client and the activities subsumed under the category of the relevant professional group, such as medical and surgical procedures.

ICD-10 is one of the means of measuring progress towards the goal of health for all. The incidence and prevalence of major diseases and related health problems are determined by means of its internationally recognized terms. The use of classifications is thus related to measurement in health care, and the important recent development of a classification scheme for nursing practice is intimately related to the issue of measuring nursing.

The development and measurement of the quality of clinical outcomes are important recent trends that affect developments in clinical nursing management. The quality of care is the subject of one of the European targets for health for all *(3)*. Particular attention is paid to clinical outcome quality through continuous quality development *(4)*. This is a dynamic process using the best outcomes of care continuously to raise the overall quality of care. The evaluation of quality development includes measuring progress in the clinical outcomes of nursing.

The emerging information society is the third important recent development that pertains to the issue of measuring nursing. Electronic records of patient care and computerized clinical databases have been introduced. The use of information technology for the storage, retrieval and communication of data has accelerated the development of information systems that capture essential data on care by means of minimum basic data sets. Such key data sets are particularly important in monitoring the development of clinical quality. Recognizing the importance of measuring progress in improving health and the quality of care, the WHO Regional Office for Europe has taken an active interest in promoting the development of information systems *(4)*. Measuring nursing implies registering or capturing by electronic means data on nursing care that are produced as a result of the documentation of clinical practice.

This chapter describes both the potential to gain information about nursing practice that is offered by classifications and high-level instruments for measuring clinical outcome quality, and the realization of this potential through the use of telematics applications for registering data.

Measurement in theory

The use of classifications is linked to the qualitative measurement of nursing through the use of a nominal scale: a scale of names. The desire to measure clinical outcomes in order to monitor quality can be seen as linked to quantitative measurement of nursing through the use of ordinal, interval or even ratio scales to express the amounts to be measured.

Measuring nursing means assigning numbers to the objects of nursing *(5)*. Numbers can indicate the kinds and amounts of the characteristics possessed by the objects. Measuring nursing can thus be of at least two kinds:

- qualitatively assigning numbers to the objects of nursing on the assumption that they represent the kinds of characteristics possessed by the objects; and

- quantitatively assigning numbers to the objects of nursing on the assumption that they represent the amount of the characteristics.

From a systematic point of view, these two kinds of measurement can be seen as levels in a hierarchy. From the lower to the higher levels, the scales of measurement are nominal, ordinal, interval and ratio. Nominal scales are used to measure nursing qualitatively by means of numbers indicating an object's membership in one of a set of exhaustive and mutually exclusive classes. Ordinal, interval and ratio scales are used to measure nursing quantitatively.

In measurement by nominal scale, objects are placed into categories according to defined properties. Applied to the international classification of nursing practice, this means classing patients' conditions into categories of nursing diagnoses according to their clinical characteristics. Thus, a condition with the clinical characteristics of breathing with discomfort and increased effort, shortness of breath, nasal flaring, changes in respiratory depth, the use of accessory muscles, altered chest excursion and fremitus is classed as dyspnoea. Diagnostic categories such as dyspnoea are represented by numbers and the numbers assigned to clinical conditions represent membership in a category. For example, the category dyspnoea might be assigned the number 15. Measuring nursing qualitatively means using numbers as category names, for labelling only; the numbers have no quantitative meaning.

Measurement by ordinal scale assigns numbers to objects according to the rank order of a particular attribute. It may be regarded as ranking objects in quantitative categories according to the relative amounts of the specified attribute. In addition to being able to categorize and rank objects at the ordinal level, one can also order objects according to the size of their numerals and the relative size of the differences between two objects, but such a scale, called an interval scale, has no absolute zero point. Ratio-level measures give all the information provided by interval measures, but they have points at which zero represents an absolute absence of the relevant attribute *(5)*.

Evaluating quality development requires measuring progress in the clinical outcomes of nursing. This appears to require scales to rate the status of the patient condition, because a change in status is hoped to express the outcome of nursing interventions *(6)*. The condition of the client in relation to the objective and subjective characteristics of nursing diagnoses (such as breathing with discomfort and increased effort, shortness of breath, nasal flaring, changes in respiratory depth, the use of accessory muscles, altered chest excursion and fremitus) should thus be rated on a scale of the following type:

1 = the clinical characteristics are extreme
2 = the clinical characteristics are severe
3 = the clinical characteristics are moderate
4 = the clinical characteristics are minimal
5 = there are no clinical characteristics.

A rating of dyspnoea that moves from 1 to 5 expresses a significant change in the status of the condition, and might therefore reveal an increase in clinical outcome quality with regard to dyspnoea as a result of nursing interventions.

Deciding whether to measure nursing by a classification on a nominal level or by rating scales measuring on ordinal or interval level is no trivial matter. Depending on the level of measurement, fundamentalists claim only specific statistical techniques are available. Only non-parametric statistics are considered appropriate with lower-level measures, i.e. nominal and ordinal scales. Parametric statistics are only permissible with higher-level measurements, i.e. interval and ratio scales. On the other hand, pragmatists claim that there are no clear distinctions between levels of measurement and that therefore the nature of the research question should direct the choice of statistical operation, not the level of measurement *(5)*.

Important recent developments in nursing – the use of classifications and the continuous development of clinical outcome quality – are thus linked to different levels of measuring nursing. Measuring nursing, however, is more than a question of using classifications or going beyond them to higher levels of measurement. It also implies registering or capturing data produced as a result of the measuring process. The potential for the provision of information on nursing by using classifications or other measures will be realized in the twenty-first century through the development and implementation of clinical telematics applications for nurses.

Measurement in practice

International classification for nursing practice

The need for an international classification for nursing practice was first proposed to ICN at the Council of National Representatives in 1989. Through a resolution, the Council asked member associations to take part in describing classification systems for nursing care, information systems and data sets. The resolution was referred to the Professional Services Committee. An advisory group has since been appointed including Norma Lang of the United States, Randi Mortensen of Denmark and June Clark of the United Kingdom as consultants and Margaret Murphy and Madeline Wake of the United States and myself as technical advisers. The development of a classification can be described in three steps: collecting terms, grouping them, and establishing a hierarchy within the group. The final product can be described as a pyramid of concepts. The top of the pyramid – the top term of the classification – is the most general concept. The bottom of the pyramid – the lowest-level terms of the classification – comprises the most specific concepts. An example from outside nursing might illustrate the idea (Fig. 1).

Fig. 1. Pyramid of concepts

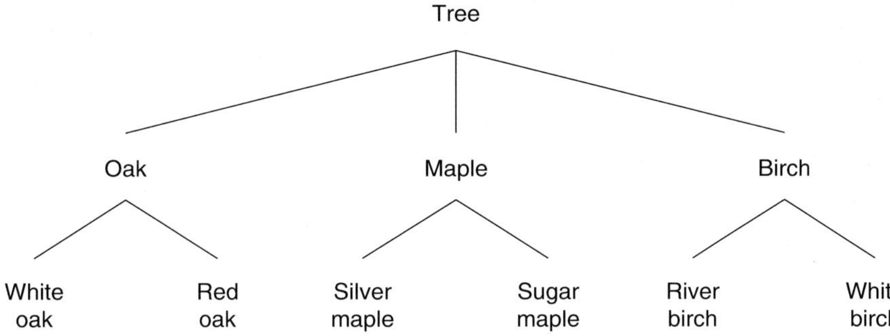

Tree

Oak | Maple | Birch

White oak | Red oak | Silver maple | Sugar maple | River birch | White birch

Source: Nielsen & Mortensen *(7)*.

Like the three major pyramids of ancient Egypt near Cairo, ICNP consists of an arrangement of three pyramids of concepts, describing:

- nursing phenomena supplementary to existing classifications of, for example, diseases, handicaps, disabilities and impairments;
- nursing interventions supplementary to, for example, medical and surgical interventions; and
- the clinical outcomes of nursing efforts.

Building pyramids is a huge task. As a first step, ICN and its advisory group made an international survey to identify possible health-related classifications in nursing. The terms of these classifications might be looked on as the building blocks of the three pyramids of ICNP. In a second step, Randi Mortensen and I undertook the task of developing an architecture for classifications of both nursing phenomena (nursing diagnoses or problems) *(7)* and nursing interventions or activities. This architecture was presented at the sixth meeting of the advisers in June 1995. At a meeting in the autumn of 1995 with technical advisers Madeline Wake and Amy Coenen, this architecture was further refined and the outline of two pyramids of concepts is emerging. The third pyramid – nursing-sensitive outcomes – still lacked an architecture as of January 1996. In parallel with the more technical work of the advisers, the idea of ICNP has been presented to nurses all over the world to initiate a consensus process. ICN held meetings in collaboration with national nurses' organizations in the Americas in 1993, Africa in 1994 and Asia in 1995. In Europe, the EU research and development programme will partly finance two meetings to promote the idea of ICNP as part of a project called TELENURSE, which is led and coordinated by Randi Mortensen *(8)*. These meetings will be open to all nurses interested in the idea of a common professional language. Besides the events at the European level, similar activities are to be organized at the national level.

ICNP is meant to supplement traditional health indicators of mortality and morbidity with measurable health indicators related to clinical nursing, by adding measurable nursing aspects to the concept of health embodied by WHO in its policy for health for all *(3)*. Ideally, ICNP will allow nursing to be measured in three dimensions:

- the diversity of patient populations from a nursing point of view (nursing diagnoses or problems);
- the variability of practice patterns (nursing interventions); and
- the variations of clinical results (outcomes).

Of course, this type of information about nursing practice promises to have great potential for influencing health policy by making nursing practice measurable in an internationally recognizable way. This will make nursing visible in a new and forceful manner.

This invites the idea of a European database on nursing and health *(8)*. A database structured according to ICNP would allow Europe-wide descriptions of the diversity of patient populations from a nursing point of view, the variability of practice patterns and the clinical results of care. A European database comprising essential data on nursing care would supplement traditional mortality and morbidity indicators with measurable health indicators related to clinical nursing. In the long run, this could influence EU policy and add nursing aspects to the concept of health in the WHO European policy for health for all.

Establishing a European database on nursing and health along the lines of ICNP is a task worthy of the efforts of WHO collaborating centres in the European Region, in alliance with nurses in government. A preliminary step in this task is the development of nursing databases on the national level. The goals of the ICNP project *(2)* include: "To achieve utilization of ICNP by nurses at country level for development of national databases". This work can be seen within the context of the demand for continuous quality development of clinical practice in the health care sector in Europe.

Continuous quality development in clinical outcomes

In 1993, the WHO Regional Office for Europe, in collaboration with the Danish Ministry of Health and National Board of Health, proposed a national policy for continuous quality development *(4)*. Its elements include the development of information systems capturing essential data on care through the creation of minimum data sets, and the establishment of clinical databases for monitoring progress towards the goal of health for all.

As mentioned, the Regional Office has taken an active interest in promoting the development of information systems. Two such systems have been introduced in recent years. WHOCARE focuses on surgical wound infections and DIABCARE on the quality of care of diabetes. A similar system is under development: the ORATEL computerized information system for quality management in oral health *(4)*.

Faced with the rapid appearance of several isolated national clinical databases based on personal computers (PCs), dealing with medical specialties such as breast cancer and hip fractures, the Danish Board of Health in 1993 created a small working group to describe *(9)*:

> a set of principles for the development, establishment and exploitation of such electronically supported clinical databases in order to ensure that developments of databases for monitoring clinical quality would be integrated and coordinated with other developments of information systems within the Danish health care system. In particular the integration of isolated PC-based clinical databases with emerging electronic patient records was considered essential in order to avoid double registration of the same clinical data.

A description of the nursing module of databases for monitoring clinical quality included in the guidelines of the National Board of Health was based on the use of the emerging ICNP to structure data on nursing care *(9)*. In accordance with these guidelines and the proposed national policy, the Danish Institute for Health and Nursing Research has since been developing a database on nursing phenomena, i.e. diagnoses or problems, interventions and outcomes, since adequate information systems must include essential nursing care data *(10)*.

The success of nursing interventions in terms of clinical outcome can be measured as the degree to which nursing has succeeded in alleviating or relieving patients' problems. Fig. 2 illustrates this type of measurement, using the rating scale, set out above (see p. 244).

From both theoretical and practical points of view, measuring the continuous quality development of clinical outcomes in nursing offers new challenges, as one can move beyond the mere use of classifications

Fig. 2. Rating of clinical outcome in nursing: dyspnoea

Dyspnoea: BEFORE Clinical characteristics	Rating 1	 2	 3	 4	 5
Breathing with discomfort	X				
Breathing with increased effort		X			
Shortness of breath		X			
Nasal flaring	X				
Changes in respiratory depth		X			
Use of accessory muscles	X				
Altered chest excursion	X				
Fremitus		X			
Dyspnoea as a whole		X			

EVALUATION

INTERVENTION

Dyspnoea: AFTER Clinical characteristics	Rating 1	 2	 3	 4	 5
Breathing with discomfort			X		
Breathing with increased effort				X	
Shortness of breath				X	
Nasal flaring		X			
Changes in respiratory depth					X
Use of accessory muscles				X	
Altered chest excursion					X
Fremitus					X
Dyspnoea as a whole				X	

Source: Nielsen *(10)*.

to higher levels of measurement. The value of these measures, however, lies ultimately in their capacity to supply information about the bad and good results of clinical nursing practice.

Unfortunately, the capture of the results of measurements of clinical outcome quality in nursing is restricted by the possibilities of collecting basic information. The problem is the lack of uniform and standardized data sets required for the surveillance of people's needs for nursing care and the measurement of clinical outcome.

Nurses must contribute to the establishment of a European structure for health information. As part of an information society, nurses should take part in the development of telematics applications to measure nursing. Such applications should capture the data produced by measuring nursing practice with classifications or other means.

This is the rationale behind two projects initiated by the Danish Institute for Health and Nursing Research and partly financed by the EU research and development programme for telematics in health care: TELENURSING *(8,11)* and TELENURSE *(12)*. Both projects have been concerned with promoting the development of telematics applications designed to register and organize data describing the quality of clinical practice in nursing as seen from the viewpoint of the profession.

TELENURSE: telematics applications for nurses

To found the development of patient-oriented information systems for nursing practice in the nursing process – that is, clinical realities as seen by professional nurses – the Danish Institute for Health and Nursing Research formed a consortium in 1991 to apply for funds from the European Community programme on advanced informatics in medicine. The consortium members hoped that the project could be the start of computer-based clinical research in Europe to continue the WHO project on people's needs for nursing care *(13)*.

The project proposal was not, however, accepted. Instead, the European Commission launched concerted action on nursing and invited delegates to a preparatory workshop in Brussels in June 1992. Participants from Belgium, Denmark, France, Greece, Ireland, Italy, the Netherlands, Portugal, Spain and the United Kingdom presented proposals on the subject of nursing. Randi Mortensen, Director of the Danish Institute for Health and Nursing Research, was elected leader of the action. An agreement was reached on a draft work plan *(14)* whose original title was "Concerted action on telematics for nursing: European classification on nursing practice with regard to patient problems, nursing interventions and patient outcomes, including educational measures". The project later received the practical name of TELENURSING, but the original title was an early attempt to introduce ICNP to a European audience of nurses.

TELENURSING focused on nursing problems or diagnoses, interventions and outcomes for two reasons. First, they are incorporated into ICNP. Second, the development of clinical information systems and databases on nursing in Europe should be built around the three axes of ICNP to encourage the Europe-wide comparability of essential data on nursing care. Nurses from EU countries, Norway and Slovenia took great interest in TELENURSING.

TELENURSING ended in December 1994. In response to a call for proposals from the EU research and development programme on telematics applications for health care, the Danish Institute for Health and Nursing Research submitted a project proposal called TELENURSE *(12)*. The TELENURSE consortium comprised partners from 11 countries, and its proposed project was among those retained for funding.

The total project budget amounts to about ECU 100 000. The evaluators unexpectedly recommended that TELENURSE focus on promoting consensus on the use of ICNP in Europe. The TELENURSE consortium was thus required to set aside funding for two European consensus conferences, to be held in Greece in 1996 and Portugal in 1998. These meetings are open to all nurses interested in a common professional language. Besides the events at the European level, the Commission required parallel activities to be organized at the national level. Partners of the TELENURSE consortium are thus requested, as part of the project, to translate a first version of ICNP into their languages (Danish, Dutch, Finnish, French (Switzerland), German, Greek, Italian and Portuguese) and organize national meetings promoting the idea of ICNP as a common classification to be used in Europe. Other partners may well join the project, such as nurses from Slovenia. In addition, TELENURSE was presented at a conference on health informatics held in Bucharest in 1995.

TELENURSE represents a unique opportunity to involve the European Region in the development of ICNP. This is related to the second goal of the ICNP project: to achieve recognition by the national and international nursing communities *(2)*.

Furthermore, TELENURSE is about the development of nursing modules for electronic patient records. TELENURSE is part of a group of EU projects addressing this topic, and thus provides a unique opportunity for field testing the first version of ICNP as a common framework for documenting nursing care electronically.

The main task is to promote consensus on ICNP, an associated minimum data set for nursing and a structure for nursing data. To support the consensus-building process, TELENURSE will include the development of simple prototypes illustrating possible uses of ICNP.

In particular, TELENURSE will address the need for structured and standardized clinical nursing data in telematics applications used by nurses working in hospital wards or in primary care, as well as nurse managers, health care administrators, policy-makers and clinical researchers. The term clinical nursing data means data organized according to the nursing process on nursing problems, interventions and outcomes.

When analysed, data on care from clinical nursing record systems will provide what has been missing until now: information on the quality and cost–effectiveness of nursing care. TELENURSE will promote the use of ICNP by enabling existing clinical nursing record systems to record, store, access, process and communicate countable and comparable data derived from clinical nursing practice. As a long-term goal, this will allow the data to be used for various purposes, including local clinical audits and more global research-oriented analyses of practice. The data used for daily clinical practice can be recycled for the long-term monitoring of quality if clinical databases and patient records are integrated and compatible. Fig. 3 shows the cyclical flow of data to different user groups and applications that is envisaged in the TELENURSE project.

TELENURSE will use this cyclical flow of data in small-scale demonstrations of the use of ICNP in:

- terminology work
- electronic patient records
- clinical databases
- nursing minimum data sets.

A number of systems for recording clinical nursing data are in operation in hospitals throughout Europe. The strategy of the TELENURSE project is to strengthen rather than replace them. The demonstrators will therefore take the form of add-on modules or other modifications to existing systems.

Data entry will be approached in two ways at the demonstration sites. One will be the library approach; new libraries of interventions

Fig. 3. Cycle of data flow: TELENURSE

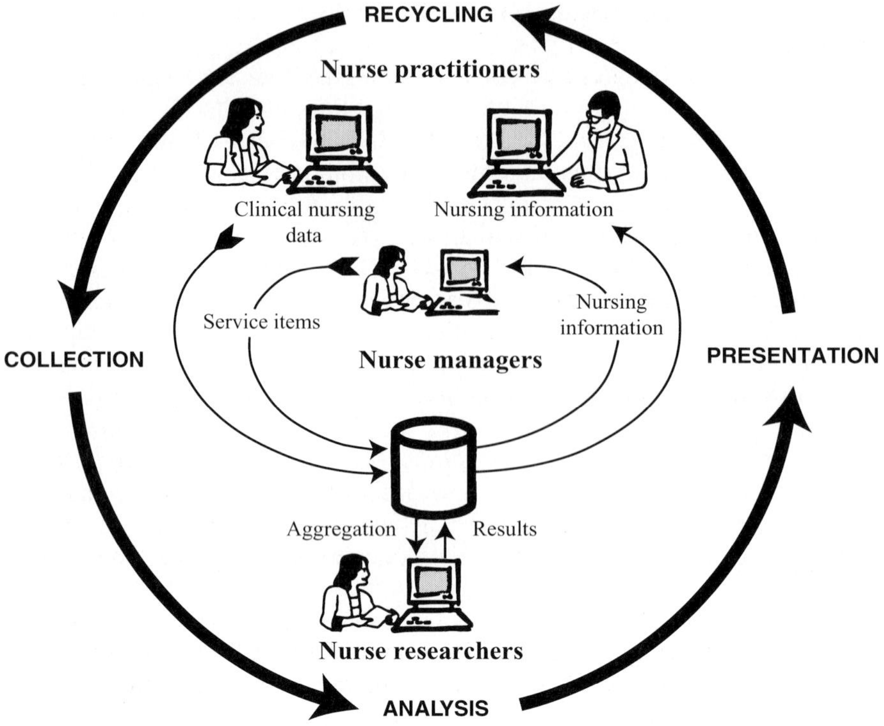

Source: TELENURSE *(12)*.

will be constructed at all sites to conform to the need for structured and standardized data in a minimum data set for clinical nursing. Second, the compositional approach will be applied to data entry. In addition, data display and manipulation facilities will be strengthened, both to accommodate the use of structured and standardized data and to improve the usability and user acceptance of nursing record systems.

One of the strategic objectives of TELENURSE is to prepare for the development of a European database on nursing and health built on electronic sampling of comparable data on nursing care in different European countries. TELENURSE will promote the use of ICNP by presenting an adequate design for the storage of data on clinical nursing care and a tool for the analysis of the data collected. The results of analyses will be fed back to nurses and health care managers by means of a presentation tool to be demonstrated in the project.

A clinical nursing database will be created primarily to store data collected from operational nursing record systems at different sites in a number of European countries. Data will be collected using a minimum data set derived from ICNP and subdivided into problems, interventions and outcomes. It will also be made comparable to the emerging ICNP.

The prototype analytical tool will allow the analysis of data in terms of nursing problems, associated interventions and their outcomes. The statistical analyses to be performed on data will range from elementary frequency counts to advanced analyses of associations and causal relations. These analyses will be used for the monitoring and surveillance of nursing care, quality assurance and planning and resource management.

The widespread introduction and use of clinical nursing record systems will depend on the improvement of their clinical appropriateness. TELENURSE will address this issue in relation to the use of standard clinical data sets, classifications and terminology organized around problems, interventions and outcomes. It will also be addressed in the clinically oriented extensions that will be developed within the project.

The ultimate goal of TELENURSE is the evaluation of nursing activities by measuring nursing: registering structured data to produce information that might support the development and improvement of clinical quality and cost–effectiveness in nursing care.

In sum, the emergence of ICNP, the continuous development of clinical quality in nursing and the growing use of electronic patient records to document nursing practice are all aspects of measuring nursing. Such measurement is essential if the impact of nursing care is to be documented and made visible. Today, the product of the measuring process must be captured or registered electronically. The use of telematics applications for nurses is the only means of realizing the information potential promised by the use of classifications (particularly ICNP) and other measures, and of turning these measures into an effective tool in the struggle to improve clinical care in the European Region.

THE NEXT STEP

The WHO study on people's needs for nursing care *(13)* was an early attempt to collect standardized clinical nursing data on a Region-wide level. TELENURSING was an attempt to pursue this goal by starting to develop standard data sets and classifications of nursing problems, interventions and outcomes to prepare for the use of modern information technology as a tool. TELENURSE can be seen as taking up where the WHO study left off through computer-based clinical nursing research in Europe. In the future, modern information technology will be used to measure nursing in Europe at different levels and at regular intervals. The study of people's needs for nursing care must therefore be electronically revisited.

References

1. *International statistical classification of diseases and related health problems (ICD-10). Tenth revision 1992*. Geneva, World Health Organization, 1992.
2. *Nursing's next advance: an international classification for nursing practice (ICNP) – working paper*. Geneva, International Council of Nurses, 1993.
3. *Health for all targets. The health policy for Europe.* Copenhagen, WHO Regional Office for Europe, 1993 (European Health for All Series, No. 4).
4. *Continuous quality development. A proposed national policy.* Copenhagen, WHO Regional Office for Europe, 1993 (document EUR/ICP/CLR 059).
5. Waltz, C.F. et al. *Measurement in nursing research*, 2nd ed. Philadelphia, F.A. Davis, 1991.
6. Martin, K.S. & Sheet, N.J. *The OMAHA SYSTEM. Applications for community health nursing*. Philadelphia, W.B. Saunders, 1992.
7. Nielsen, G.H. & Mortensen, R.A. Nursing terminology as a means of identifying nursing diagnoses. Basic level diagnostic categories in nursing. *Vård i Norden. Utveckling og forskning*, **4**: 5–13 (1994).
8. Nielsen, G.H. & Mortensen, R.A. TELENURSING. *In*: Laires, M.F. et al., ed. *Health in the new communications age*. Amsterdam, IOS Press, 1995, pp. 115–126.
9. *Principper for udvikling, etablering og anvendelse af databaser for klinisk kvalitet* [Principles for the development, establishment and use of databases for clinical quality]. Copenhagen, National Board of Health, 1993 (in Danish).
10. Nielsen, G.H. *Klinisk resultatkvalitet i sygeplejen: forslag til principper for udvikling, etablering og anvendelse af landsdækkende database for klinisk resultatkvalitet i sygeplejen* [The quality of clinical results in nursing: proposal for principles for the development, establishment and use of databases for clinical quality in nursing]. Copenhagen, Danish Institute for Health and Nursing Research, 1994 (in Danish).

11. NIELSEN, G.H. & MORTENSEN, R.A. *TELENURSING reports*. Copenhagen, Danish Institute for Health and Nursing Research, 1994, Vol. I–V.
12. *TELENURSE. Telematics applications for nurses. The nursing research potential of electronic health care records and the role of nursing research centres in Europe*. Copenhagen, Danish Institute for Health and Nursing Research, 1995.
13. ASHWORTH, P. ET AL. *People's needs for nursing care. A European study*. Copenhagen, WHO Regional Office for Europe, 1987.
14. NIELSEN, G.H. & MORTENSEN, R.A. *TELENURSING workplan for a concerted action in Europe on classifications for nursing practice: nursing diagnoses/problems, nursing interventions and outcomes*. Copenhagen, Danish Institute for Health and Nursing Research, 1992.

Annex 1

Declaration and Recommendations of the First WHO Meeting of Government Chief Nurses of the Newly Independent States, Almaty, Kazakstan, 30 August–1 September 1993

The following Declaration and recommendations were made by the leaders of nursing and midwifery who participated in the First WHO Meeting of Government Chief Nurses of the Newly Independent States in 1993. The countries represented were Armenia, Kazakstan, Kyrgyzstan, the Russian Federation (Tumen *oblast*), Turkmenistan and Uzbekistan, with observers from Mongolia. The Declaration was made on 1 September 1993 in Almaty, Republic of Kazakstan, and unanimously endorsed by all participants and observers.

Second Declaration of Alma-Ata

The development of nursing, midwifery and other so-called middle-level health personnel should be a priority for all countries. As the largest group of health personnel in every country, nurses play a key role in maintaining and improving the health of the population. In the past, however, the practice, training and wellbeing of nurses have been neglected and their contribution to health care has been undervalued.

We believe that this development is long overdue. It is needed today more than ever, when the health of our people is under threat because of the serious economic difficulties being faced by all the former republics of the USSR. Nursing and midwifery provide cost-effective solutions to health care problems, as shown by evidence from many countries around the world.

We recognize that each of our countries has its own unique situation, its own strengths and its own needs. Nevertheless, in our discussions we have identified a number of common issues – development needs which we all share. These needs are as follows.

Leadership

The development of nursing and midwifery is impossible without strong leadership from within the professions themselves. The positions of Chief Nurse and Chief Midwife in the ministry of health must be occupied by a qualified nurse, midwife or feldsher, and supported with appropriate staff and budget. Where no such positions exist, they should be created as soon as possible.

The process of nursing reform

A group of leaders should be convened under the leadership of the Chief Nurse to lead the reform process and advise the government. This group should work closely with the Republic Council for Nurses and Midwives.

National action plans

Each country should develop a national action plan for nursing, as recommended by the 1992 World Health Assembly. This plan should be endorsed and actively supported by ministries of health.

The national action plan for each country should address the following key issues:

- a legal and regulatory framework for nursing;
- the authority, responsibilities and role of senior nurses in *oblasts* and hospitals;
- a professional structure for middle-level personnel, clarifying each grade's role and functions;
- the education and training of middle-level personnel at basic, post-basic and continuing levels, and its reorientation towards primary health care;
- the development of professional associations.

The socioeconomic position of nurses

The professions cannot develop their potential without improvements in salaries and working conditions. Measures should be taken by governments to "care for the carers".

Resources

Funding should be made available by ministries of health for nursing development. In addition, they should actively seek funding from international agencies and other donors.

International links

Nurses in all our countries want closer international links in order to exchange ideas and experiences. Links should be strengthened with other NIS, with other countries outside the NIS and with the World Health Organization. The WHO collaborating centre for primary health care and nursing, Almaty, Kazakstan, will continue to play a leading role in maintaining these networks.

Recommendations to countries

Participants and observers from Armenia, Kazakstan, Kyrgyzstan, Mongolia, the Russian Federation (Tumen *oblast*), Turkmenistan and Uzbekistan will undertake the following activities:

1. publicize the Second Declaration of Alma-Ata as widely as possible;
2. inform ministries of health and nursing and midwifery colleagues about the results of this meeting, including the Declaration and recommendations;
3. continue the development of a national action plan for nursing and keep WHO informed about progress;
4. continue the development of the LEMON (LEarning Materials On Nursing) project and maintain regular contact with the project coordinator;
5. maintain regular contact with the Nursing and Midwifery unit, WHO Regional Office for Europe, and supply it with information about country needs, developments and potential projects;
6. maintain regular contact with other participants in other NIS;
7. participate in the Second Meeting of Government Chief Nurses of the Newly Independent States in 1994 and encourage other NIS to participate.

Recommendations to WHO

[WHO should:]

1. publicize as widely as possible the Second Declaration of Alma-Ata;
2. write to ministers of health in all participating countries, drawing their attention to the Declaration and recommendations, and asking them to support the development of a national action plan for nursing as outlined by participants from their country;
3. circulate the meeting report to participants and ministers of health as soon as possible;

4. continue the development of the LEMON (LEarning Materials On Nursing) project and maintain contact with each country;
5. strengthen the collaboration between the WHO Nursing and Midwifery unit, and other relevant WHO programmes at [the Regional Office] and headquarters, and in each participating country;
6. help countries to network with each other and to become more active members of the international nursing community;
7. organize the Second WHO Meeting of Government Chief Nurses of the Newly Independent States in 1994.

Annex 2

Statement and Recommendations of the Second WHO Meeting of Government Chief Nurses of the Newly Independent States, Bishkek, Kyrgyzstan, 24–26 August 1994

The statement by participants and observers was unanimously adopted at the close of the meeting. The countries represented were Kazakstan, Kyrgyzstan, the Russian Federation (Ministry of Health and Tumen *oblast*), Tajikistan, Turkmenistan and Uzbekistan. The participants also adopted the following recommendations.

Statement

We hereby reaffirm the Second Declaration of Alma-Ata on nursing in the newly independent states, adopted at the First WHO Meeting of Government Chief Nurses of the Newly Independent States in 1993. In addition, we express our commitment to implementing WHO policy on the role of the nurse, recognizing that the policy is relevant to all health professionals with a nursing function or orientation, be they nurses, midwives or feldshers. This policy describes the nurse's key functions as follows:

- providing and managing nursing care, whether promotive, preventive, curative, rehabilitative or supportive, to individuals, families or groups;
- teaching patients, well people and health care professionals;
- acting as an effective, equal member of the health care team;
- developing nursing practice through critical thinking and research.

Recommendations to countries

[Countries should:]

1. inform ministries of health and nursing colleagues about the results of this Meeting, wherever possible using the media (journals, television, radio, etc.) to encourage debate about nursing;

2. work on the development of a national action plan for nursing as part of national health policy (the term national is understood to refer to each country as a whole and not to any ethnic group or other entity);
3. establish, or where appropriate enlarge, the nursing department in each ministry of health, appointing a full-time salaried post of Chief Nurse and other specialist nursing and/or midwifery posts within the ministry according to priority health needs;
4. provide learning materials on nursing in local languages through implementation of the WHO LEMON project by country LEMON groups, and maintain regular contact with the WHO project coordinator;
5. review, update and translate into local languages the WHO country nursing and midwifery profiles;
6. strengthen the network of NIS nursing leaders, using the WHO collaborating centre for primary health care and nursing in Kazakstan and the proposed WHO collaborating centre for nursing, Moscow, Russian Federation, wherever appropriate;
7. maintain regular contact with the Nursing and Midwifery unit, WHO Regional Office for Europe, and keep it informed about successes and needs;
8. review the current terminology used to describe middle-level health workers, and where appropriate devise suitable new terminology in keeping with WHO policies.

Recommendations to WHO

[WHO should:]

1. publicize the results of this meeting as widely as possible, using the media whenever appropriate, including communication with ministries of health;
2. assist countries to provide learning materials on nursing through implementation of the LEMON project, maintaining regular contact with each existing country LEMON group, and encouraging new LEMON groups to be formed in all CCEE/NIS which do not yet participate in the project;
3. continue collaboration between the Nursing and Midwifery unit and other relevant WHO programmes at [the Regional Office for Europe] and headquarters, and in each country;
4. continue dissemination of WHO materials in Russian, especially the translation of the book *Nursing in action*;[1]

[1] Copenhagen, WHO Regional Office for Europe, 1993 (WHO Regional Publications, European Series, No. 48)

5. assist NIS nursing leaders to make links with nursing leaders from other countries in the Region and worldwide;
6. work with nursing leaders in Sweden to organize the Third WHO Meeting of NIS Government Chief Nurses in Stockholm in 1995.

Annex 3

Statement and Recommendations of the Fourth WHO Meeting of European Government Chief Nurses and WHO Collaborating Centres for Nursing and Midwifery, Glasgow, United Kingdom, 18–20 October 1994

Participants and observers from 32 Member States of the WHO European Region unanimously adopted a statement at the close of the Fourth WHO Meeting of European Government Chief Nurses and WHO Collaborating Centres for Nursing and Midwifery. The statement details challenges to nursing, and the participants made recommendations to countries and WHO to propose some ways of tackling them.

Statement

We hereby reaffirm the relevance of the 1988 Vienna Declaration on Nursing in Support of the European Targets for Health for All, and the recommendations from the WHO European Conference on Nursing, 1988. We believe that these statements continue to provide a vision to guide the development of nursing[1], and practical proposals to strengthen the contribution of the Region's five million nurses and midwives to health for all.

We believe that the role of the health for all nurse[2], as outlined in the Declaration, is to help people throughout their life span, as individuals,

---

[1] Nursing is used here as a general descriptive term. Terminology and definitions vary from country to country, and the term nurses should be understood to include all health workers doing nursing-related work, including nurses, midwives and feldshers. For brevity, reference is made throughout to nurses and nursing.

[2] The health for all nurses is one who contributes to achieving the goals of health for all. The mission, role and functions are comprehensively described in the Vienna Declaration and subsequent WHO publications, notably SALVAGE, J., ED. *Nursing in action. Strengthening nursing and midwifery to support health for all* Copenhagen, WHO Regional Office for Europe, 1993 (WHO Regional Publications, European Series, No. 48).

families and groups, to determine and achieve their physical, mental and social potential, and to do so in the context of the environment in which they live and work. This requires nurses to develop and perform functions that promote and maintain health as well as prevent ill health. Nursing also includes the planning and giving of care during illness and rehabilitation, and encompasses the physical, mental and social aspects of life as they affect health, illness, disability and dying.

However, major political, economic and social transformations are taking place in the Region and indeed worldwide. As leaders of change we acknowledge the resulting need to take account of them, recognizing that each of our countries has its own unique situation, strengths and needs. Within this changing environment, both old and new health care needs must be met in new ways, and health services must respond more sensitively to those needs. A number of special challenges to nursing must therefore be tackled – and at all levels, from individual to international.

The challenges to nursing

[The challenges to nursing include:]

- influencing health care reform to ensure a continuing commitment to equity and social justice, especially for vulnerable groups and those in greatest need;
- supporting the positive trend towards nurses working in partnership with individuals, families and groups, acting as patient/client advocates, and stimulating community empowerment in health care;
- developing national action plans for nursing as part of health plans and playing a full part in formulating national health policy, thus securing the necessary commitment and resources for nursing development for better health;
- strengthening the links between nursing inputs and health outcomes through increasing the effectiveness and efficiency of nursing practice, by means of critical thinking and research, and better collection and use of relevant data for monitoring and evaluation;
- promoting dialogue with the public, policy-makers and other health care personnel in order to clarify how nursing can maximize its contribution to health in a multiprofessional setting;
- empowering effective leadership in nursing, paying special attention to the development of women leaders;
- making better use of all available sources of influence, especially networks and alliances within and beyond the nursing community.

Recommendations to countries

[Countries should:]

1. promote dialogue about nursing using all available means, including the media, and inform nursing colleagues, ministries of health, budget holders, other health personnel and the public about the results of this Meeting and about the vision and mission of the health for all nurse;
2. recognizing the continuing relevance of WHO policies and guidelines, and the international leadership provided by the Nursing and Midwifery unit [at the Regional Office for Europe], encourage health care leaders, policy-makers and donor agencies to use WHO guidance and to seek WHO input on nursing development programmes;
3. ensure that the professional and corporate contribution of nursing leaders is recognized and encouraged in ministries of health and other appropriate national institutions;
4. ensure that nurses and midwives have the basic, postbasic and continuing education they need to help them to become effective practitioners, teachers, managers, researchers and leaders, and the opportunity to make appropriate use of their skills and knowledge;
5. strengthen the links, and promote concerted action, between government chief nurses, national nursing and midwifery associations, regulatory bodies, WHO collaborating centres for nursing and midwifery, and other health care leaders;
6. take active steps to utilize WHO collaborating centres for nursing and midwifery as sources of expertise and creativity in health and nursing development, and as advisers to governments and other health care leaders and institutions;
7. provide high-quality materials on nursing in local languages, for example, through translation and widespread dissemination of WHO publications such as *Nursing in action* and the LEMON (LEarning Materials On Nursing) package;
8. maintain regular contact with the Nursing and Midwifery unit [at the Regional Office for Europe] and contribute to the country nursing and midwifery profiles and analysis of nursing and midwifery in Europe;
9. take part in the Fifth WHO Meeting of European Government Chief Nurses.

Recommendations to WHO

[WHO should:]

1. publicize the results of this Meeting as widely as possible;
2. prepare a mission statement on nursing for circulation to countries and to intergovernmental and nongovernmental organizations to affirm the continuing relevance of the Vienna Declaration and to reinforce the nursing response to newly emerging key issues in health;
3. continue to promote close and active cooperation between the Nursing and Midwifery unit and other relevant WHO programmes in headquarters, the Regional Office and countries, ensuring that nursing and midwifery development is appropriately resourced by the Organization;
4. encourage the development of nursing leadership in the newly independent states of the former USSR through cooperation with health care institutions in Sweden to organize the Third WHO Meeting of Government Chief Nurses of the Newly Independent States in 1995;
5. maintain and strengthen links with government chief nurses, WHO collaborating centres for nursing and midwifery, and other networks and provide help in the development of national action plans for nursing;
6. prepare a comparative analysis of nursing and midwifery in Europe and develop indicators of nursing development at national level, taking due account of related global initiatives, in order to stimulate progress and to help implement [World Health Assembly] resolution WHA45.5 on strengthening nursing and midwifery in support of strategies for health for all;
7. help countries to provide high-quality materials on nursing through advice on translation and dissemination of relevant WHO publications such as *Nursing in action* and the LEMON package;
8. plan the Fifth WHO meeting of European Government Chief Nurses, including WHO collaborating centres for nursing and midwifery, and paying special attention to relationships with other health care disciplines.

Annex 4

Statement from the Third WHO Meeting of Government Chief Nurses of the Newly Independent States, Stockholm, Sweden, 17–21 June 1995

The following statement was made by the leaders in nursing and midwifery who participated in the Third WHO Meeting of Government Chief Nurses from the Newly Independent States. The participants came from: Armenia, Azerbaijan, Belarus, Estonia, Georgia, Kazakstan, Kyrgyzstan, Latvia, Lithuania, the Republic of Moldova, the Russian Federation, Tajikistan, Turkmenistan, Ukraine and Uzbekistan.

Statement

We, the participants, hereby unanimously affirm the Second Declaration of Alma-Ata on nursing in the NIS (1993). The principles and issues highlighted in the Declaration continue to be relevant to the countries which drew up the Declaration, and are also affirmed by the other NIS which are participating in this Meeting for the first time. They can be summarized as follows.

The development of nursing and midwifery should be a priority for all countries. As the largest group of health personnel, nurses play a key role in maintaining and improving the health of the population. In the past, however, the practice, training and wellbeing of nurses have been neglected and their contribution to health care has been undervalued.

We believe that this development is long overdue. It is needed today more than ever, when the health of our people is under threat because of the serious economic difficulties being faced by all the republics of the former USSR. Nursing and midwifery provide cost-effective solutions to health care problems, as shown by evidence from many countries around the world.

We recognize that each of our countries has its own unique situation, its own strengths and its own needs. Nevertheless, we have identified a number of common issues – development needs which we all share. These are as follows.

Leadership
The development of nursing and midwifery is impossible without strong leadership from within the professions themselves. The positions of Chief Nurse and Chief Midwife in the ministry of health must be occupied by a qualified nurse, midwife or feldsher and supported with appropriate staff and budget. Where no such positions exist, they should be created as soon as possible.

National action plan for nursing
Each country should develop a national action plan for nursing as recommended by the 1992 World Health Assembly. This plan should be endorsed and actively supported by ministries of health.

Nursing education
The basic and continuing education of nurses and midwives needs reforming and orienting towards health and primary health care. This should result in professionals who work competently and independently rather than as assistants to doctors.

The Nursing Declaration of Alma-Ata was reaffirmed at the Second WHO Meeting of Government Chief Nurses of the Newly Independent States, held in Bishkek, Kyrgyzstan, 24–26 August 1994. The Bishkek statement also expressed commitment to implementing WHO policy on the role of the nurse, recognizing that the policy is relevant to all health professionals with a nursing function or orientation, be they nurses, midwives or feldshers. This policy describes the nurse's key functions as follows:

- providing and managing nursing care, whether promotive, preventive, curative, rehabilitative or supportive, to individuals, families or groups;
- teaching patients, well people and health care professionals;
- acting as an effective, equal member of the health care team;
- developing nursing practice through critical thinking and research.

We, the participants at the Third WHO Meeting of Government Chief Nurses of the Newly Independent States, wish to renew our commitment to the Second Declaration of Alma-Ata and the Bishkek statement. In addition we would like to emphasize three issues which underpin the process of change now under way, and which are the key to our future success in improving the quality of health care. These issues are as follows.

1. We acknowledge the vital importance of human relationships, networks and mutual learning in our change process. Our countries' traditional emphasis on formal, centralized authority needs to shift to more informal, cooperative, non-competitive ways of working which are more appropriate to our current needs and desires.
2. We believe that attitude changes are the key to successful change, and that these can best be encouraged and developed in nursing by focusing on participative leadership and education reform. These initiatives should be led by nurses themselves, but should also involve other health professionals and the public.
3. We acknowledge the value of external help from WHO and other agencies and governments in this change process. However, we wish to emphasize that such help should be led by us and our countries, working in partnership with these helpers. This requires a major shift away from market/provider/professionally-led initiatives and systems which foster dependency, towards needs-led ones based on mutuality. This echoes the spirit of health for all. It also reflects both the need to reorient health care systems away from narrow professional concerns towards those of society, and the current efforts to develop nurse–patient relationships which place the client at the centre of our concerns.

Annex 5

Participating in international meetings

International meetings are an exciting and important way of exchanging ideas, information and support. We in the Nursing and Midwifery unit of the WHO Regional Office for Europe have learned from experience, however, that a meeting of people from different cultures can easily lead to misunderstandings and frustration. Thus, in WHO meetings, it helps us to follow a few simple rules; perhaps you will find them helpful too. They are relevant whether you are making a formal speech or participating in a discussion.

Language

Even if simultaneous translation is provided at the meeting, many people will be using a language that is not their mother tongue. To enable people to understand you as fully as possible, speak slowly and clearly; use short sentences and avoid difficult technical terms or idiomatic expressions. To be sure that you understand others, do not hesitate to ask speakers to repeat or clarify their words; if you did not understand, other people probably did not understand either.

Giving a talk or a report

When people are listening to a talk or a report in a foreign language, they need more time to absorb it. When you speak, take your time, and allow pauses between each main point. Remember that people easily become tired when using a second language, so keep the talk short. A logical structure for the talk will also help comprehension. If you are describing a case study or other specific examples or data from your own country, outline the main points and principles, but do not give too much detail. Remember that simple stories about people translate more vividly and are more memorable than descriptions of organizational structures or abstract theories.

Using interpreters

If your talk is being translated simultaneously, give the interpreter a copy of the paper or a list of the main points in advance. He or she will appreciate having a short discussion with you beforehand, especially if he or she has no special knowledge of the subject matter. Many terms do not have an exact equivalent in another language and this can lead to misunderstandings in translation; the word nurse is a good example of this.

If your talk is being interpreted by someone who translates every few sentences (consecutive interpretation), remember that it takes twice as long as simultaneous translation. If you have been given 30 minutes on the programme, your talk should actually last only 15 minutes.

Audiovisual aids

Overhead transparencies, slides and handouts can all be very useful ways of reinforcing your message. If you decide to use these aids, however, keep your material short and simple. Avoid the temptation to fill your slide or transparency with small writing, complicated diagrams and lots of information; use it for headlines and key points only. Before you give your talk, check with the organizers that the equipment you need is available, and that it works.

Visual messages such as cartoons, photos or simple diagrams can all be very effective for an international audience, and help to keep the tone relaxed and communicative. If your talk is being translated, ask in advance for your overheads to be translated too. (It is always useful to take spare overheads and pens with you, just in case.)

Let's communicate!

A final word of encouragement: the purpose of our meetings is to communicate. People communicate best when they say what they believe, as simply and as directly as possible. Your listeners will respond to this and it will help to make your talk memorable and enjoyable for both you and them.

Annex 6

Running small group meetings

All meetings, even short discussions in small groups, are complex human interactions. To ensure the best results, the content needs to be clear and well expressed, and the process must be well conducted. The climate must be open and friendly, and any difficult feelings or conflicts must be dealt with appropriately. All these things have to be managed at the same time, usually by the group leader or facilitator. It is hard for one person to pay attention to all these things, so it is better to share the responsibilities; for example, one person keeps time, another takes notes, and a third chairs the discussion.

Fig. 1 shows the main strands that are present in any meeting, even if they are not always recognized or given due respect: the technical content, the process or procedure, and the emotions, feelings or group dynamics. If the purpose of any meeting is developmental – in other words, to help the participants move from their present position (point A) to a new position (point B) – the facilitator must ensure that the different strands are managed effectively.

Fig. 1. Group discussion: helping participants move from

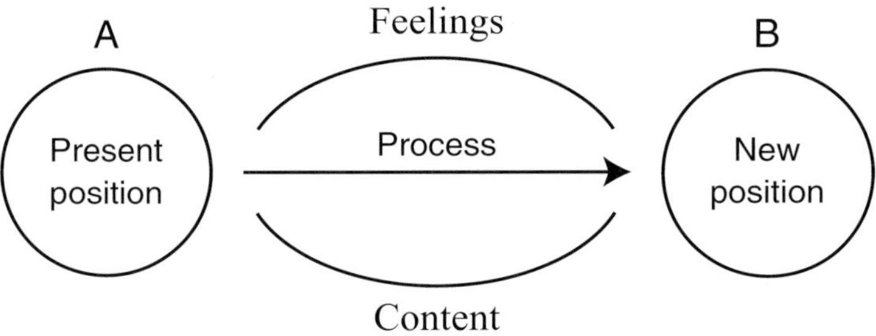

Group leader's or facilitator's responsibilities

1. Before the session starts, arrange the room – and the chairs, preferably in a circle or around a table – and ensure the temperature is comfortable.
2. When you begin the session, ask the participants to choose a chairperson or to confirm they are willing for you to chair it.
3. If the group is required to make a report, ask for a volunteer to be the rapporteur or note taker. If no one volunteers, choose someone yourself.
4. If the group is small enough, ask the members to introduce themselves briefly. Stop them gently if they take up too much time.
5. Make sure everyone understands the purpose of the session, and any outcomes that are expected (such as a verbal report to a plenary session, or a summary on paper of the main conclusions). Remind people that they do not need to take notes, as the group's conclusions will be recorded; it is difficult to concentrate on a discussion and take full notes at the same time.
6. Ensure that the session starts and finishes on time.
7. Make sure everyone participates; if necessary, ask people who have already spoken to keep quiet and give the others a chance. Resist the temptation to fill in silences yourself.
8. Encourage people to speak directly from their own experience, as well as contribute theoretical points. Allow them time to express themselves properly, but not to make long speeches; this is a discussion session.
9. Make sure people speak clearly and loudly enough for everyone to hear.
10. Ensure that the group's task is completed in time. It is best to end the discussion five minutes early, to enable the rapporteur to give feedback.

Rapporteur's responsibilities

1. Ensure that you understand what kind of report is needed, such as a verbal report to a plenary group, a summary on a flip chart or an overhead transparency.
2. Record the main points of discussion only; it is impossible and unnecessary to write down everything that is said.
3. Record the main points on a large sheet of paper, such as a flip chart, for everyone to see and check during the session.
4. Check with the group five minutes before the end of the session to ensure that you have recorded the main points accurately, and to give people a chance to correct or add points.
5. Give the report to the plenary session, after inviting your group members to add or amend anything they wish.

Group members' responsibilities

1. Make sure you have completed any preparatory work you were asked to do in advance of the session.
2. Be there on time.
3. Make sure you understand the purpose of the session and the expected outcomes.
4. Participate actively, contributing from your theoretical background as well as from your experience. Avoid making speeches, however; this is a discussion, not a lecture.

Annex 7

Fund-raising: a simple guide

Here is an eleven-step guide to fund-raising.

1. Make a plan

A group of colleagues involved in trying to raise funds and other support for your project should meet to make a work plan for this activity. Allocate responsibilities, set deadlines and review progress regularly.

2. Set your targets

Decide together what help you need. Do you want money, or would you like other kinds of support? It is quite acceptable to ask potential donors for support in kind, such as office equipment for your project (a fax machine or computer, for example), help with tasks such as printing and translation, free use of an office, or staff such as voluntary workers and secretaries. Many organizations cannot give much money, but can provide other types of help.

3. Prepare your proposals

Prepare a menu or list of proposals, ranging from small to large. You can divide the major activities into phases, and request separate funding for each. Many donors like to test the water by funding the first phase and evaluating the results before deciding whether to invest in the next. Use the WHO guide entitled *Writing a funding proposal – it's as easy as 1, 2, 3*[1], available in English only from the WHO Regional Office for Europe. Look at examples of successful proposals prepared by other projects. The proposal document should include:

---

[1] Geneva, World Health Organization, 1986 (document WHO/HMD/NUR 86.2)

- a rationale or explanation of why the project is needed;
- a description of what you hope to achieve and the specific impact on health;
- a description of the activities proposed; and
- a detailed budget with the estimated costs of all the proposed activities.

The costs include administration, translation, transport and other hidden costs, as well as the costs of workshops, publications, etc.

4. Prepare background materials

Compile a range of materials to support your proposal(s). This could include LEMON brochures and newsletters, letters of support from organizations such as WHO or the health ministry in your country, and information on or a profile of nursing in your country.

5. Identify potential donors

Ask the WHO Liaison Officer (if your country has one) or the health ministry to tell you what foreign or international organizations or agencies are based in your country or have a special interest in it. Some countries have directories of these organizations, or clearing-houses in the health ministry or elsewhere. There are many types of potential donor, including:

- international agencies, such as WHO, UNICEF and the World Bank;
- foreign governments (approached through embassies and local project offices, for example);
- foreign nongovernmental organizations;
- your own government; and
- ocal businesses and charities.

6. Gather information about donors

Use formal and informal sources, networking and gossip to find out what you can about potential donors. Find out their priorities and regulations, and their needs, such as those for publicity.

7. Approach donors

Use the phone, mailings, exploratory meetings with individual donor agencies or groups, and contact with visitors from other countries to approach donors. Do all this before you send them your detailed proposals.

8. Prepare targeted proposals

When you have done all these things, you will be ready to write more detailed proposals for the donors who have shown an interest and explained their priorities and available funds to you. You must tailor your proposals to their priorities. Also, clarify with them what you are prepared to offer in return, especially if the potential donor is a commercial organization seeking public recognition of its sponsorship of your project.

9. Financial management

In anticipation of all the money you are going to receive, find out how you can set up a bank account. In the CCEE and NIS, regulations controlling banking and hard currency are often confusing and may create obstacles. Some countries impose high taxes on foreign income and some may even freeze the money so you cannot use it. Find out the safest and most flexible option for your project. Sometimes international or United Nations agencies are willing to look after your money. Appoint a treasurer, perhaps trustees: people with some expertise in finance, business or accounting whom you can trust to give you good advice. Make sure that all cheques or other payments are approved by two people and keep scrupulous records of every transaction.

10. Publicize the donation

Success breeds success; when you receive a donation, tell everyone. Publicity is good for the project and the donor, and for the image of nursing. Also, donors like to invest in projects that they think will be winners. A small donation for your project could be seen as seed money and might encourage bigger donations.

11. Manage the donation

Once you have the money, you must remember your responsibility to account to the donors and to the project steering group for everything that is spent and every activity undertaken. Keep up a regular dialogue with donors to maintain their interest in your project and to avoid misunderstandings.